The Politics of Size

The Politics of Size

Perspectives from the Fat Acceptance Movement

Volume I

Ragen Chastain, Editor

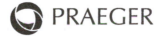 PRAEGER

AN IMPRINT OF ABC-CLIO, LLC
Santa Barbara, California • Denver, Colorado • Oxford, England

Copyright © 2015 by Ragen Chastain

Library of Congress Cataloging-in-Publication Data

The politics of size : perspectives from the fat acceptance movement / Ragen Chastain, editor.
    2 volumes ; cm
    Includes bibliographical references and index.
    ISBN 978–1–4408–2949–9 (hard copy : alk. paper) — ISBN 978–1–4408–2950–5 (ebook)
1. Overweight persons—Health and hygiene. 2. Overweight persons—Social conditions.
3. Overweight persons—Psychology. 4. Fat-acceptance movement. I. Chastain, Ragen, editor.
RC552.O25P64   2015
613.2′5—dc23   2014014311

ISBN: 978–1–4408–2949–9
EISBN: 978–1–4408–2950–5

19 18 17 16 15   1 2 3 4 5

This book is also available on the World Wide Web as an eBook.
Visit www.abc-clio.com for details.

Praeger
An Imprint of ABC-CLIO, LLC

ABC-CLIO, LLC
130 Cremona Drive, P.O. Box 1911
Santa Barbara, California 93116-1911

This book is printed on acid-free paper ∞

Manufactured in the United States of America

This anthology is dedicated to Judi Richardson (aka Josephine Cranberry). Judi passed soon after she completed her piece for this anthology. Judi was a force within the Fat Acceptance movement—in her own words, she "attended several conventions, retreats, put on workshops, participated in pickets of antifat businesses, marched to support the cause, and partied hearty at the dances." She also started the SAFE meetings that continue in LA to this day. But Judi was also engaged in another form of activism—living her life large and in charge, refusing to be held back by the prejudice that works to keep fat people from making our dreams come true. Judi passed away surrounded by her friends and she is, and will continue to be, missed.

Thank you Judi, for showing so many of us the way and helping to create a movement. We all benefit from your work and will move forward in your honor and try to do you proud.

Contents

INTERSECTIONAL EXPERIENCES

INTRODUCTION

Perspectives on Perspective

Ragen Chastain

When I was approached by Praeger to create this anthology I was thrilled. I knew immediately that I wanted to put together a work that truly explored as many perspectives as possible from the Fat Acceptance movement. I set out to create an anthology that was intersectional in its scope, including People of Color, Queer people, people with disabilities, diverse ages, women, men, and Trans* people, and including pieces written by those inside and outside of academia.

Much of the stigmatizing, shaming, and oppression that fat people experience is based on stereotyping. In truth fat people are as diverse as any group of people who share a single physical characteristic. There are fat athletes, fat couch potatoes, fat people of every political and religious affiliation, disabled fat people, fat PhDs, fat Queer people, fat People of Color, and we go about the business of fighting our oppression in myriad ways. My goal with this anthology is to give you the opportunity to hear from and about as many of those people and types of activism as possible.

In a world where people ignore and ridicule actual fat people but clamor to hear about the experiences of celebrities in fat suits, and where government task forces are formed to "deal with the problem of obesity" without even one obese person included, where People of Size are talked about and talked at, but all too often not heard, I endeavored to take every opportunity to create a platform for People of Size to talk about our experiences. If you are a regular reader of anthologies, you'll definitely find pieces that are familiar to you, fully researched and written in the language of academia. You'll also find first-person accounts of what it's like to be part of the Fat Acceptance movement. I've edited the pieces as little as possible to let the authors' voices shine through, preferring to give readers a diverse collection of authentic voices and working hard not to sacrifice that authenticity for consistency.

I encourage you to read with an open mind, and to remember that any feelings of disbelief or defensiveness are places to dig deeper, to check privilege, and to remember that we are each the best witness to our own experiences, welcome to ours.

I

Express Yourself: Fat Activism in the Web 2.0 Age

Cat Pausé

The Internet is an amazing place—it allows for people to access information at the tips of their fingers. It enables individuals to form, maintain, and grow relationships. It may foster democracy and open communication between disparate parties. As a fat person, the Internet allows my mind to have regular exposure to fat positivity and my body to have access to fashionable clothing. And, as a fat person, the Internet allows anyone who is so inclined to climb into my living room and remind me how disgusting they find me. The Internet giveth and the Internet taketh away.

One appeal of the Internet for me is the Fat-o-sphere—a community of fat-positive people who support one another.[1] There are individuals all over the world who are engaged in fat-positive work, and many of us have developed relationships over the years. I feel connected to these individuals, most of whom I have never met in person, and confident that if I were to call on them for help, they would rally around me. In the Fat-o-sphere, you can find fashion advice, sex tips, and friendship.

Many individuals in the fat community are taking advantage of the Internet for the purposes of social justice. The Internet allows for a range of diverse people to share their voice, their story, and their perspective with a global community. It also allows them to promote campaigns, engage others in their cause, and find similar-minded people to collaborate with. Especially useful for social activism are Web 2.0 tools. Web 2.0 tools are ones that allow the information user to also become an information producer.[2] Web 2.0 tools include blogs (hosted on platforms like WordPress and BlogSpot), microblogs (hosted on platforms like Twitter and Tumblr), and social media platforms such as Facebook. These tools have allowed for activists around the world to connect, engage, and change the larger discourse.[3]

What's great about Web 2.0 is that it allows for everyone (with a computer and access to the Internet) to have a voice—open participation, if you will. And it allows for marginalized groups to push back against the normative discourse. In this way, social media is the perfect way to situate oppositional fat politics online.[4] Most of the mainstream discourse around fatness centers on concerns about the obesity epidemic. Individuals of all sizes are regularly told that being fat is unhealthy, that fat people are miserable, and that inside every fat person is a thin person who really wants to be set free.

Through the use of social media, a different story about fat is emerging. Fat people are able to contribute to the larger discussion on fatness. They are able to tell their stories, share their views, and often contradict the normative messages. Tumblrs like "Exciting fat people" highlight fat individuals who are doing exciting things. The Stocky Body Image library allows for a visual representation of fat people with heads doing a variety of everyday things;[5] it is an alternative to the headless fatty usually used in the media to accompany stories about fatness.[6] The Size Diversity Task Force has collected videos of fat people[7] sharing their stories of medical discrimination; these videos are available for viewing for a range of purposes: to educate medical professionals, to challenge the layperson's understanding of evidence-based care, to eliminate the feeling of isolation other fat individuals may feel.

There are many different ways to use Web 2.0 for fat activism. You can choose to be spectator—reading, watching, and engaging with the work of others. I spent months lurking around fat-positive blogs and Tumblrs; reading, listening, watching. I remember listening to the Two Whole Cakes Fatcast[8] with Marianne Kirby and Lesley Kinzel with a goofy smile on my face. Here were two fat women, talking about topics and issues that were relevant for my fat life. I learned a great deal from listening to their conversations; especially about the language I could use to describe my own experiences and feelings about how the world treated my fat body.

The next level of engagement would be slacktivism. This term has been coined to define the activism that consists of liking something on Facebook, or changing your profile picture to symbolize your support of a cause. The name stems from the lack of work it takes to be involved in this kind of activism, but there are strong arguments to be made for the impact it may have.[9] In fat activism, especially, sharing a fat-positive article, or liking a fat-positive page, or changing your profile pic to a fat-positive picture; exposing your friends and family to anything fat positive may make a huge difference both in how they think about fat people, and also how they think about themselves.

My first forays into fat activism were slacktivism masked behind my work as an academic. I would post academic pieces on my Facebook page that challenged the dominant narrative around fatness. I would mention the research

I was doing on weight identity in fat women. In this way, I was able to introduce pieces of fat activism into my online world in a way that felt safe for me. As an academic, I could share these articles with a nod and an "Interesting dialogue—thoughts?" attitude. I engaged in this academic slacktivism for over a year. Then, one day, after giving it a great deal of thought, I updated my status to read, "Cat Pausé is proud to be a fat feminist who works for social change."[10] As I've written about previously, taking this step required a great deal of courage and reflection on my part—who proudly identifies as a fat person? Of course, looking back on that now, I smile fondly at that version of myself—who was so afraid of that baby step into activism.

My next step was creating a fat-positive Tumblr. Tumblr hosts microblogs, and integrates a dashboard so users may follow each other and be exposed to the contents of each other's Tumblrs (similar to the Facebook Newsfeed). Most of a person's time on Tumblr is spent either posting or scrolling. I began a Tumblr, wanting a place to collate fat-positive material. I began following other fat-positive Tumblrs, and soon my dashboard was filled with positive representations of fatness: pictures, stories, quotes, and links to articles and blogs. Many people host multiple Tumblrs, each focusing on a different area of interest. Until recently, I maintained only one, and I love the multimedia aspect of the platform. I also love how Tumblr allows for activist projects to go viral.

For example, Brian Stuart of Red No 3 began a campaign to respond to the children's book *Maggie Goes on a Diet*.[11] The book tells the story of Maggie, a fat girl who is unhappy. In the book, Maggie demonstrates many stereotypical fat behaviors, like late-night binging and not wanting to participate in sport. Maggie is also bullied in the book. By the end of the book, Maggie has lost weight and is now one of the popular kids. In his work, Brian created cover art for alternative Maggie stories, including "Maggie Goes on Friend of Marilyn"[12] and "Maggie Reclaims the Word Fat." In creating alternative covers for Maggie stories, Brian pushed back against the dominant narrative. In his imaginings, Maggie is a fat girl who embraces who she is. In some of his versions, Maggie herself is involved in fat activism. Stuart's use of Tumblr to revise Maggie is exactly the kind of oppositional politics that Web 2.0 tools may foster.[13] These images were reblogged across Tumblr, with each new addition restarting the cycle anew. Two years later, they still sometimes run across my dashboard. Such is the power of Tumblr.

After I maintained my Tumblr for several months, I decided to try my hand at a proper blog. Many of the authors in this collection have blogs; some maintain multiple blogs on different topics. I had always been inspired by the work of Ragen Chastain (*Dances with Fat*),[14] Kath Read (*Fat Heffalump*),[15] Kate Harding (*Shapely Prose*),[16] and many others. I was hesitant to add my voice to the mix; I wasn't sure if I had anything valuable to say, or if anyone would be interested in reading what I did have to say. On my blog, I made a conscious decision to remain on message; I write only about fatness. I felt it was important to have a consistent theme for the blog both for myself and for my readers. My other concern was about the commitment it might take to maintain a blog. As an academic, writing is something I am expected to do—but for publications in peer-reviewed journals, not online media. I decided to post once a month, on the fifth of every month. This allowed me both a schedule to stick to and a sense of control over the time commitment I would give to my new project. Now that I've been blogging for almost two years, I really love it. It allows me the space to write in a casual way that it not encouraged in academic writing. And I've begun to argue that my blog should be considered an aspect of my scholarship. Academics are slowly starting to catch on to what activists have known for years: blogging is a valid way to disseminate information, engage with others, and promote social justice. Arguments are being made to allow consideration for online work to be given credence and value within an academic career.[17] Shortly after setting up my blog, I also set up a Facebook page for my brand, Friend of Marilyn.

Besides allowing for brands, or individuals with public profiles, to have pages that represent their work, Facebook allows for the gathering of groups under umbrella topics. I belong to several Fat Groups on Facebook. These groups are a place where individuals may exchange information, engage in conversation, and share media.[18] Within a Group, an individual member may post photos, links to outside web content, and their own opinions. Facebook Groups are a space designed for small-group engagement. Anyone can create a Group—and Groups may be open (meaning anyone may join) or closed (only those invited or accepted may join). Some Groups, like Fat Studies or Big Fat World, are organized around a broad topic. Others, like Flying While Fat, have a specific purpose—to share information, opinions, and experiences on a specific phenomenon (in this case, tips and tricks for fat people utilizing air travel).

I was never going to join Twitter. I already had Facebook, Tumblr, and my blog; I had no interest in picking up another piece of social media. Twitter is a platform that allows real-time communication and information sharing through tweets. Tweets are limited to 140 characters, and tweeters are able to speak directly to another tweeter, or pull someone else into their tweet, by including that person's handle. Information may also be organized around hashtags. A hashtag is a word or phrase that is preceded by the symbol #. Some use Twitter simply to promote their blog or web page, but some use it to engage with others around issues of fat activism. Twitter allows for real-time conversations to occur between individuals all over the world. Notably, these conversations take place in public and anyone else can join in. Occasionally, a hashtag will be created by someone in the fat activism community—one of my favorites is #notyourgoodfatty. Started by @fatbody-politics and @mazzie, #notyourgoodfatty is used when a fat activist on Twitter writes about engaging in activities that are frowned upon by society; things that fat people are not supposed to do. It may be used when wearing a bikini, or refusing to order a salad; I suggested that I was done spending hours clothes shopping with straight sized friends in stores that refuse to dress my fat body. Tweeting has also become a common way to build a brand. Linda Bacon,[19] an academic who helped to develop the Health at Every Size paradigm, uses Twitter as a way to promote her work in the media. She has more than 6,500 individuals following her on Twitter. Dr. Bacon chooses not to retweet anyone else—if she shares a link or a thought or a piece of advice, it is under her own handle, @LindaBaconHAES. She also never includes others into her tweets by their handle, which may diminish the opportunity for conversation, and denies the producer of the content she is promoting the chance to be easily discovered by those who follow Bacon. Many fat activists use Twitter as a way to promote their blogs and other online writings. Some link their Twitter account to the Tumblr account, and both to their Facebook page. This way, they are able to post something on one platform and have it reposted on their other social media pages.

Another way to engage in activism through social media is by publishing in online magazines and journals. I have published several pieces in *The Conversation*, an online magazine from Australia. What I love about magazines like *The Conversation* is that they have stories on the same topics and subjects you find on the evening news—but all of the content is produced by academics that provide a scholarly context for the story. When I write an article for *The Conversation*, I prepare my piece with a theoretical foundation and integrate scholarly evidence.[20] It offers an opportunity for scholars to take our skill sets (integrating and synthesizing large amounts of science) and apply them for the purpose of social justice. And like blogging, it is increasingly being recognized as a valid form of scholarship.

One of the strengths of activism through social media is the immediacy that you are afforded when working in an instant print environment. Unlike an academic article, which can take years from conceptualization to publication, a tweet, blog, or Tumblr post can be published instantly. Another strength of Web 2.0 is the ability to bring together people from around the world—whether to collaborate on a project, organize an event, or respond en masse to an act of oppression. Living in New Zealand, I am geographically removed from the fat activism hubs of Australia, the UK, and the Bay Area in California. But social media allows me to both be aware of what is going on with fat activism and participate. For example, on a recent quiet Sunday afternoon, Associate Professor Geoffrey Miller tweeted, "Dear obese PhD applicants: if you don't have the willpower to stop eating carbs, you won't have the willpower to do a dissertation #truth."[21] Not surprisingly, many people responded to his 140 characters of fat shaming. He deleted the tweet, apologized, and soon after changed his Twitter account to protected (you had to follow him to see his tweets). A screenshot of the tweet continued to circulate, however, and social media activism sprung up around the world. Many, like The Fat Chick, responded with blog posts addressing the tweet.[22] Others retweeted the screenshot and posted it to their Facebook wall. Some sent e-mails to his department chair, demanding action and accountability for the role he plays in graduate admissions.

For my part, I considered how best to address the situation using social media. I decided that I was not interested in writing to him, or his boss, or doing anything that specifically was about him and his fat-hating tweet. I do not want to spend my time talking about how one person is fat hating; I want to spend my time talking about how our entire culture is fat hating. But his tweet does highlight a common hateful belief about fat people: that fat people are fat because they lack the willpower to be slim. And his tweet is in the context of higher education, one of the many sectors in which fat people face discrimination. As a fat woman with a PhD, I am very aware of the overt and covert ways that the education section excludes fat people.

I decided that I wanted to develop a gallery of photos of fat people with PhDs.[23] I sent out calls for help on Twitter, Tumblr, and Facebook. I also emailed a Fat Studies listserv that I subscribe to. I asked for people to send, via e-mail, a photo, along with their name, degree, and awarding institution. My requests were quickly picked up by people in the Fat-o-sphere with a higher profile than mine, like Kath Read, Marilyn Wann, and Ragen Chastain. The response was overwhelming. Within the first two days, I had received information from more than 100 individuals. The Tumblr I created, "Fuck yeah! Fat PhDs," garnered more than 300 followers and 150 pictures of rad fatties with graduate degrees, and has received a fair amount of media coverage—all of this less than a week after the offending incident. Such is the power of Web 2.0.

Engaging with social media, like any Internet engagement, is limitless; the possibilities and opportunities are never ending. There are other online venues I engage with: my Academia.edu page provides a Facebook of sorts for my academic colleagues, my YouTube channel provides a way to showcase my work in the media in a single location, and my podcast on iTunes allows people around the world to listen to my fat-positive radio show. Each individual has to evaluate what forms of Web 2.0 are most useful for them in their own personal social justice work. I find that each medium of social media I engage in allows for my work to be seen by a wide range of individuals—and also allows me to present my work in different voices. In my blog it's me as a fat person; in my Twitter it's me as a fat feminist; in The Conversation it's me as an fat academic; in Tumblr it's a mix of all three. While the tone may vary based on venue, the message is always the same: fat people deserve the same rights and dignity as nonfat people. And I am grateful that Web 2.0 tools give me so many different ways to promote my form of social justice; come and find me sometime in cyberspace!

NOTES

1. Kate Harding and Marianne Kirby, *Lessons from the Fat-O-Sphere: Quit Dieting and Declare a Truce with Your Body* (New York: Penguin, 2009), 35.

2. Michael Martin, "Social Media: Changing the Nature of Activism?," National Public Radio, online interview, April 9, 2012, http://www.npr.org/2012/04/09/150286291/social-media-changing-the-nature-of-activism.

3. Rob Procter et al., "Adoption and Use of Web 2.0 in Scholarly Communications," *Philosophical Transactions of the Royal Society A: Mathematical, Physical and Engineering Sciences* 368, no. 1926 (2010): 4039.

4. Richard Kahn and Douglas Kellner, "New Media and Internet Activism: From the 'Battle of Seattle' to Blogging," *New Media & Society* 6, no. 1 (2004): 5.

5. Lauren Gurrieri, "Stocky Bodies: Fat Visual Activism," *Fat Studies: An Interdisciplinary Journal of Body Weight and Society* 2, no. 2 (2013): 197.

6. Charlotte Cooper, "Headless Fatties," *Charlotte Cooper* (blog), 2007, http://charlottecooper.net/publishing/digital/headless-fatties-01-07.

7. Size Diversity Task Force, "Medical Advocate Project," *The Fat Chick* (blog), 2013, http://www.thefatchick.com/The_Fat_Chick/SDTF_MD.html.

8. Lesley Kinzel and Marianne Kirby, *Two Whole Cakes Fatcast*, podcast audio, 2011, http://fatcast.twowholecakes.com/.

9. Mark Pfeifle, "Changing the Face(book) of Social Activism," *Huffington Post*, June 14, 2012, http://www.huffingtonpost.com/mark-pfeifle/social-media-political-activism_b_1594287.html.

10. Cat Pausé, "Live to Tell: Coming Out as Fat," *Somatechnics* 2, no. 1 (2012): 42.

11. Paul Kramer, *Maggie Goes on a Diet* (Eagle, ID: Aloha, 2011), 7.

12. Brian Stuart, "Maggie Goes on Friend of Marilyn," *Tumblr*, October 19, 2013, http://red3blog.tumblr.com/post/11651700740/maggie-goes-on-friend-of-marilyn-okay-so.

13. Kahn and Kellner, "New Media and Internet Activism, 5."

14. Ragen Chastain, "And Size Acceptance for All," *Dances with Fat* (blog), October 15, 2012, http://danceswithfat.wordpress.com/2012/10/15/and-size-acceptance-for-all/.

15. Kath Read, "Why I Take No Shit from Anyone in My Online Spaces," *Fat Heffalump* (blog), May 28, 2013, http://fatheffalump.wordpress.com/2013/05/28/why-i-take-no-shit-from-anyone-in-my-online-spaces/.

16. Kate Harding, "Don't You Realize Fat Is Unhealthy?," *Shapely Prose* (blog), June 20, 2007, http://kateharding.net/faq/but-dont-you-realize-fat-is-unhealthy/.

17. Douglas Powell, Casey Jacob, and Benjamin Chapman, "Using Blogs and New Media in Academic Practice: Potential Roles in Research, Teaching, Learning, and Extension," *Innovative Higher Education* 37, no. 4 (2012): 1.

18. Nick Pineda, "Facebook Tips: What's the Difference between a Facebook Page and a Group?," *The Facebook Blog*, February 25, 2010, http://www.facebook.com/blog/blog.php?post=324706977130.

19. Linda Bacon, *Health at Every Size: The Surprising Truth about Your Weight* (Dallas, TX: BenBella Books, 2010), 50.

20. Cat Pausé, "Moving Beyond Weight: Why the Focus on Size Is Bad for Health," *The Conversation*, March 30, 2012, https://theconversation.edu.au/moving-beyond-weight-why-the-focus-on-size-is-bad-for-health-5903.

21. Geoffrey Miller, "Dear obese PhD applicants: if you don't have the willpower to stop eating carbs, you won't have the willpower to do a dissertation #truth," *Twitter*, June 2, 2013, http://twitter.com.

22. Jeanette DePattie, "Dear Dr. Terrible Your Bigotry Is Showing," *The Fat Chick Sings* (blog), June 2, 2013, http://fatchicksings.com/2013/06/02/dear-dr-terrible-your-bigotry-is-showing/.

23. Cat Pausé, "Fuck Yeah! Fat PhDs," *Tumblr*, June 3, 2013, http://fuckyeah fatphds.tumblr.com/.

2

Fierce Fat Fashion

Cathy Miller

Fat fashion *is* fat activism. Do you doubt it? Forget "mainstream" fashion catalogs—just look at 99.9 percent of the so-called plus-size clothing catalogs. Not a fat person in sight! Clothing for big bodies modeled on little bodies. The message is: we are completely disenfranchised, basically invisible, of little value—aesthetic or otherwise.

Clothes that you feel comfortable in, feel elegant in, feel downright alluring in are a statement that we are here, we want to be seen, and we demand to be seen. Before you can put yourself out there, you must begin to like what's underneath the clothes, love what you've got. Before you get into your clothes, *wear your body* with pride. Celebrate your body! Be proud to stand out so that your fat sister who sees you thinks, "Wow! She looks great! I'm about her size, I'd probably look great in that, too!"

You're reading this book, so you've likely heard the "Love Your Body" message before. But have you taken the steps to actually do it? The very best way is to strip naked and gaze at yourself in a mirror. Move, dance, play as you watch yourself. No comparisons, pretend you're on a desert island completely alone. So, what's wrong with the body you've got? What's not to like? Soft curves, a feeling of comfort, abundance, expansion. It's a body that you couldn't live without and you can live within. It's a body that takes you through every single day, precious beyond anything you own.

Does it take time? Yes. Sometimes, a very long time. A terrible wall of prejudice rises up and pushes against our feeling good about our bodies in our culture. We see, hear, and encounter this prejudice (and ignorance) everywhere, from our own families, our doctors (if we even go), all forms of media, self-appointed food police, on-air scolds. The mantra and message ad nauseam is to be dissatisfied with your body—even to hate it—no matter what your size. And what a vested interest it is, with the U.S. diet industry alone up to $60 billion and counting. If you add in the beauty and cosmetics industry

($53 billion), the weight loss surgery sector ($30,000 average per surgery), it's almost impossible not to internalize fat hatred. So, yes, it can take a very long time to deconstruct and overcome chronic dissatisfaction with and frustration about your body's size and shape.

So, what can help you in the quest to learn to love your body? Since this is a chapter about fat fashion, I'll be brief. Read fat-positive and body-positive literature. Definitely use the Internet—the size diversity movement is a very strong presence on the Web. Your local library will also have size-positive books; see the end of this chapter for a short bibliography.

Surround yourself with positive images of differently sized large bodies. Mainstream media has so few positive images of fat people, and so many images that denigrate fat people, that it's easy to feel invisible. Positive images *can* be found with some effort and you will be amazed at how much they help reinforce your good feelings about your body. Revel in the wonderful, sensual art of Botero and Rubens. Delight in the art of Beryl Cook. Gaze with pleasure on Leonard Nimoy's *Full Body Project* (book and online) and "The Adiposity Project" (online). Discover also *Women En Large: Images of Fat Nudes*, photographs by Laurie Edison, text by Debbie Notkin. Sculpture and other three-dimensional fat-positive art are surprisingly common and can be found at Voluptuart, an on-line store offering many forms of fat-positive art and gifts. (See the bibliography at the end of this chapter for the books and websites mentioned here.)

Remember, too, that the Internet is an incredible source of all things fat positive, including fat fashion. On the 'Net you'll find quite a gathering of members of the size-positive fat community. Forums, blogs, dating services, products, and, in my opinion, the best fat fashion out there. More on this as we go along. Also on the Web, you'll find a bouquet of "fatshionista" pages, which may have started out as one website but have become such a part of the online fat fashion scene that the word has been added to the fat-positive lexicon. Click on any link that comes up with a "fatshionista" search and you'll be regaled with numerous photos of all sizes of fat women in a dizzying array of fat fashion. You'll also discover all the photos of themselves that fat women have uploaded. So you know you're seeing bodies like yours in clothes that make the women wearing them feel terrific. Here you'll see and discover anything you'd care to know about fat fashion. I promise you'll get a huge portfolio full of new and wonderful ideas. Looking at these terrific photos has most definitely broadened my fashion world and introduced me to styles (and places to shop) I would never have known about otherwise.

Once you begin to feel good about the body you've got, you'll find clothes shopping a far more enjoyable experience. You'll also be willing to search out and find clothes that are right for you.

Most of us know about the major large-size clothing stores like Lane Bryant, Avenue, Fashion Bug, and Catherine's, so I won't put them in my list of plus-size shopping vendors. In fact, you won't find many brick-and-mortar list-ings there, as the most variety and (in my opinion) the best styles are to be found far more consistently online. A word about these big players in the plus fashion world: have you noticed the general low quality of the clothing, com-pared with that in many of the numerous clothing stores catering to "main-stream" sizes? The clothing at Lane Bryant and others is so often made of cheap fabrics, the workmanship is poor, and durability is far less than optimal. Fat women are often buying poor-quality clothing because that is all that is offered!

Before we get very far into the shopping scene, I'm going to point out a few pitfalls specific to plus-size fashion—forewarned is forearmed and you can make active efforts to avoid them. The frustrations of poor sizing, poor quality, poor cut—all the result of fat fashion being the "orphan" of the fashion indus-try. Plus-size women deal with an abysmal lack of standard sizing; those with larger bodies, especially those above a 3X, even more so. The result of this inconsistency? Depending on the manufacturer, sometimes you wear a 2X, sometimes a 4X. Your body hasn't changed, but you must deal with the frus-tration of never really being certain a garment will fit. Add to that how ter-rible an "up-sized" garment can be—sleeve length half a foot too long, shoulder seams dropping almost to your elbows, but hips too narrow. All the result of taking a size 12 and sizing up every measurement. Both are problems and can be even worse if you like to order clothing online or from catalogs.

That said, these problems simply need to be worked around, nothing we can do about them . . . unless you make a conscious decision and effort to buy from those vendors who have more of a clue about how to design a pattern to all sizes of large. I've been buying fat fashion for decades and am happy to say that, at least, it is better today than years ago, when the selections were hideous cast-iron polyester and muumuus.

Thankfully, we now have lots of choices in a wonderful kaleidoscope of styles for fat women. Some designers are even getting hip about supersized fashion; more and more choices beyond 4X are becoming available.

Choices are so where it's at! Now I can try out Goth, sexy club wear, prom dresses, beautiful Renaissance and other costumes . . . I can make just about any fashion statement I'd care to. And, I think the more statements we make, the broader our activism. Personally, I often like to dress almost as if in cos-tume and love to play with fashion. I will try *anything* to see how I feel in it! No rules. If you like what you see, try it on. Even if at first you think it's too colorful, too bold, too sexy, too conservative, too different from what you usu-ally wear. So often fashion, dressing, and image are taken so seriously—you'll have more fun if you play with it.

You never know what you might discover! See how different styles make you feel. If a style/color/whatever promotes your power, bolsters your confidence, increases your good feelings about your body ... those are the clothes you want. And, when you wear them, you will stand out. You will be a presence, far from invisible. You will inspire your fat brothers and sisters. And, unbeknownst to you, you will surprise some "average"-weight people by their positive reaction to you. Negative reactions? You know they're out there. Walk confident and proud. You'll give off an aura of "Don't like what I'm wearing? Look at your shoes!" Powerful fat activism, in my opinion.

One more thing. Dress for yourself. I know it's next to impossible not to think about how others will see you in whatever you've chosen to wear. But, in the end, dress for yourself. If you like it, if it makes you feel good, go for it. Whether it's in fashion or out of fashion, it's in bright colors considered "gauche"—who cares?—skintight or loose and flowing, showing skin or not showing skin—whatever supports good feelings and makes you face the world proudly—wear it! Go for it. And, above all, never be hesitant to think outside what's already in your closet!

What about custom-made clothing? Too far beyond your budget, you say? Think again. There's an online company, eShakti, that makes custom plus-size clothing as well as ready-to-wear in sizes to 36. At the time of this writing, custom styling on any of their pieces is only $7.50! Their styles range from classic to retro to current trends, most of them quite appealing. I've not yet ordered from this company, but it gets numerous positive reviews from those who have.

In these difficult economic times, I understand that many reading this book may not have the latitude to shop for very much in the way of clothing. It makes shopping more of a challenge, certainly, but real bargains are out there. Many thrift stores now have separate racks for plus sizes and they disappear very quickly. I've been to my local Goodwill, Salvation Army, and a couple of other similar stores to see their selection and was surprised to find some possibilities there, all the way to 6X. Be sure also to check out flea markets in your area—plus-size clothing up to 6X is becoming very popular. In addition, various size-positive organizations run plus-size-only rummage sales; among them are Big, Fat Flea in New York City and the clothing swap put on in Los Angeles by the Size Diversity Task Force. To find these clothing events, get familiar with the fat-positive blogs and forums on the Web—if you don't have a computer, head down to your public library.

A fun and economical do-it-yourself fashion project is to buy regular T-shirts in your size (or larger) and transform them into cute tops with a pair of scissors and some creativity. Very often, the larger-size T-shirts are cut for men—wide in the shoulders and narrower in the hips. This leaves you with a high-necked top with shoulder seams that reach to your elbows and too snug around your hips. However, you'll be pleasantly surprised, even amazed, at what you can do with T-shirt "surgery." Google "T-shirt modification" to find site after site (including how-to videos) with fantastic ideas on how to make any T-shirt into something you'll love to wear. You can also find numerous books on the subject; you'll find a couple titles in the resource lists at the end of this chapter. T-shirt "surgery" is fun and it's easy.

When money is tight, you can learn to make your own clothes. A good number of plus-size patterns to size 32 are offered by the big pattern companies like Simplicity and McCall's. Some really great patterns to size 6X and even beyond are offered by smaller specialty pattern companies such as Coni's Patterns or BurdaStyle. All are easily found using any search engine.

Any discussion on sewing large sizes would not be complete without mentioning Barbara Deckert, author of *Sewing for Plus Sizes* (Taunton Press, 2002). The book is a must-have for sewing plus-size fashion; Ms. Deckert also has a blog as well as an online sewing class. This lady is a great resource.

Have you ever gone through a trendy store within the "junior" section of a large department store and seen numerous styles that, if in your size, would look great on you? Then, when you get to the "plus-size" department, far fewer items catch your eye in the same way?

I certainly have. I felt it was a downright conspiracy to keep anyone over a size 10 (and most definitely anyone over a size 4X) out of (1) really cute fashions, no matter how good they may look on a larger body, and (2) never, ever in the clothing that you could find in *both* the trendy departments and the "plus-size" department. Designers don't want it known that many of the same styles that look good on a thin body also look good on a fat body. I have a theory that fashion designers feel their clothing is "devalued" if anyone above a size 6 or so can wear and look good in their designs. In addition, if word gets out to their tiny customers that the same styles look good on larger women, these designers fear the loss of their "exclusive" clientele.

I knew how well many fashions made for smaller sizes would translate beautifully into larger sizes if only someone would try it! A few large-size fashion breakthroughs occurred over the years from the late 1980s to the 1990s, but so much more creativity was needed.

I finally got fed up waiting for someone else to provide the clothing I longed for and decided I'd take on the job. Further, making beautiful clothing for large sizes was an opportunity for direct fat activism, making a difference in the lives of fat women. So I went into the business of fat fashion design. Since my finances as well as my experience were just about nil, I knew my only chance for success would be to start small and learn as I went. I did it with $500 and three incredibly simple designs that I fashioned out of beautifully colored and patterned batik sarongs that I purchased at street fairs.

I had a part-time job and spent the rest of my time sewing those three designs at home until I had enough to take to a local fat event. When I sold out in three hours, I knew I'd really stumbled on to something. In addition to attending fat events (such as the conventions of the National Association to Advance Fat Acceptance), I created my own website and began selling online.

In three years, I quit my part-time job and went completely professional. I stopped sewing my own and had them made for me in Indonesia. In four years, I was selling many styles that I designed and had made for me in Bali, Indonesia, from the most beautiful batik fabrics I could find. And, yes, I did buy some of the cutest tops and dresses in the "junior" department, brought them to my Balinese tailors and had them make patterns up to size 6X—they worked beautifully, just as I knew they would.

If you're interested in starting your own plus-size business, I strongly encourage you to do so. You can do it! If you are a large-size person, you already know what looks good on you. That means you know something about sizing, cut, and style. This puts you ahead of 99 percent of fashion designers who have no clue how to design for large bodies. If you can sew, you are even further along to creating designs and starting your own business.

Even if you can't sew, you can still design. Try taking a draping class if your local community college offers it. At the time of publication, even YouTube offered an online class, and several how-to books are available. A draping class will teach you how to take a length of fabric and drape it on your body (or on a dressmaker's form) to create basic designs.

Think simple but creative when you first begin. The plus-size fashion scene is wide open for anything you might create. Go slow, learn as you go, and don't invest more money than you can afford to lose.

When you've got some pieces ready to sell, you can always start by putting them online on eBay or any of the handmade art "marketplace sites" websites—Etsy, Artfire, and others. Then, when you've discovered what sells and you're gaining momentum, create your own website (many free website builders are available on the Internet). Become a vendor at National Association to Advance Fat Acceptance conventions and other fat-positive events; sell at street fairs.

I began with very little money, no experience (outside of sewing my own large-size clothing), and no business plan. I created my business as I went along, not doing business by forecast or future planning but by always assessing the current needs and wants of my customers. I worked from 8 to 10 hours a day; going on the road to events was really tiring, but I thrived and so did my business. By the time I'd been in business for 10 years, gross sales were in the six digits and rising. In 2006, I sold my business and retired.

Along the way I had the opportunity several times to move into wholesale. But I was never truly interested because I so enjoyed the interaction with my retail customers. Their self-discovery, their joy and pleasure in my designs meant every bit as much to me as the profit I was making. I had joyfully tearful calls from customers telling me that after many years afraid to go to the beach or pool, they purchased a swimsuit from my company and made the plunge. Then there were the numerous husbands who called me to thank me for designs that finally convinced their wives that they were indeed beautiful women. This was fat activism to me, in a very real way—every day, for every customer as well as for myself, again and again, to reinforce the love and acceptance of our bodies, our curves, our roundness, and our beauty.

The resources I've listed are my favorites and reflect my tastes in fat fashion, fat-positive books, and other resources. There is far more out there on the World Wide Web! I strongly encourage you to do your own exploring on the search engine of your choice to discover all that is out there.

FAT SHOPPING

Asos Curve, http://www.asos.com/Women/Curve-Inspire-Size/Cat/pgecategory.aspx?cid=9577&r=2
The "Curve" department of Asos is within the more size-comprehensive website. Very cute junior clothing and accessories. U.S. sizes 14–24. Most items low to mid-range.

Decent Exposures, http://www.decentexposures.com
100 percent stretch cotton bras and underwear, custom made for all sizes. Reasonably priced.

E-Shakti, http://www.eshakti.com
Custom clothing for sizes 0–36 (6X). Mid-range pricing. Gets rave reviews from many of the Fatshionista sites.

Evans, http://evansusa.com
Cute styles, something for almost every age and taste. U.S. sizes 10–28. Many items generously sized. Mid-range prices, most under $100 but over $35. Based in the UK, much European styling.

Forever 21 Plus, http://www.forever21.com/product/Category.aspx?br=PLUS&category=faith_main
The "Plus" department of Forever 21 is within the more size-comprehensive website. Young, trendy styles for sizes XL–3X.

Juno Active, http://www.junonia.com
Activewear of all kinds in sizes 14–40. Most items priced in the mid-range.

Love Your Peaches, http://www.loveyourpeaches.com
Fashions for all occasions, for all ages. Sizes 1X–6X, generously sized.

Making It Big, http://www.makingitbig.com
More conservative styles, high quality, and beautiful fabrics. Sizes 2X to 8X. Most items in the higher end price range.

Marisota, http://www.marisota.com
   Sister company to Simply Be. Clothing somewhat more conservative,
   however still very stylish. U.S. sizes 8–28, most items generously sized.
   Pricing is mid- to high range.
OneStopPlus, http://www.onestopplus.com
   Plus fashion marketplace for many plus-size clothing stores, including
   Avenue, Lane Bryant, Woman Within, and many more. Sizes 12W–44W.
Simply Be, http://simplybe.com
   Junior styles, darling clothes, U.S. sizes 10–28, many items generously
   sized. Majority of items are priced in the mid-range. Based in UK, much
   European styling.
Torrid, http://www.torrid.com
   Young, trendy fashions for sizes 1X to 5X. Much of their clothing tends to
   run somewhat small. Low-range pricing.

FAT FASHION SEWING, PATTERNS, AND T-SHIRT MODIFICATION RESOURCES

35 T-Shirt Hacks to Try, http://skyturtle.net/11-t-shirt-hacks-totry/
BurdaStyle Patterns http://www.burdastyle.com/pattern_store/patterns?for=1
Deckert, Barbara. *Sewing for Plus Sizes: Creating Clothes That Fit &
   Flatter*. Newtown, CT: Taunton, 2002.
Deckert, Barbara. **Plus-Size Pattern Fitting & Design**. Online sewing class.
   http://www.craftsy.com/class/plus-size-pattern-fitting-and-design/133
Fashion Patterns by Coni, http://www.fashionpatterns.com/
Filian, Cathie. **101 Tees: Restyle + Refashion + Revamp**. Asheville, NC:
   Lark Crafts, 2011.
Kwik Sew Patterns, http://kwiksew.mccall.com/women-s—plus—pages
   -3023.php.
Nancy's Notions, Plus-size pattern page http://www.nancysnotions.com/
   category/patterns/plus+size+patterns.do.
Nicolay, Megan. **Generation T: Beyond Fashion: 120 Ways to Transform a
   T-shirt**. New York: Workman, 2009.
Plus-Size Sewing Blogs, http://quitereasonable.blogspot.com/2011/03/plus-
   size-sewing-blogs.html.
T-shirt Makeovers, http://pinterest.com/susanknauff/t-shirt-make-overs/.
T-shirt Surgery, http://pinterest.com/jayapratheesh/tshirt-surgery/.

"FATSHIONISTA" WEBSITES

Fat Chic: It's not about trying to look thin, http://www.fatchic.net.
Diary of a Fatshionista, http://diaryofafatshionista.com/.

FATshionista, http://pinterest.com/asiahall/fatshionista/.
Fatshionista!, http://fatshionista.livejournal.com/.
Fatshionista Pool, http://www.flickr.com/groups/fatshionista/pool/.
The Frugal Fashionista, http://frugalfatshionista.blogspot.com/.

FAT-POSITIVE BOOKS

Bacon, Linda. *Health at Every Size: The Surprising Truth about Your Weight.* Dallas, TX: BenBella Books, 2008.

Brittingham, Kimberly. *Read My Hips: How I Learned to Love My Body, Ditch Dieting, and Live Large.* New York: Three Rivers Press, 2011.

Lebesco, Kathleen. *Revolting Bodies?: The Struggle to Redefine Fat Identity.* Boston: University of Massachusetts Press, 2004.

Molinary, Rose. *Beautiful You: A Daily Guide to Radical Self-Acceptance.* Berkeley, CA: Seal Press, 2010.

Saguy, Abigail. *What's Wrong with Fat?* New York: Oxford University Press, 2013.

Wann, Marilyn. *Fat!So?: Because You Don't Have to Apologize for Your Size.* Berkeley, CA: Ten Speed Press, 1998.

Wolf, Naomi. *The Beauty Myth: How Images of Beauty Are Used against Women.* New York: Morrow, 1991.

FAT ART RESOURCES

The Adiposity Project, http://adipositivity.com/.
Beryl Cook, http://www.berylcook.org.
Edison, Laurie, and Debbie Notkin. *Women En Large: Images of Fat Nudes.* San Francisco: Books in Focus, 1994.
Fernando Botero bibliography, http://www.amazon.com/Fernando-Botero/e/B001JOC9F0.
Nimoy, Leonard. *The Full Body Project.* Brooklyn, NY: Five Ties, 2007.
St. Paige, Edward, and Edward Paige. *Zaftig: The Case for Curves.* Seattle, WA: Laughing Elephant, 2003.
Voluptuart, http://voluptuart.com/.

3

Civil Rights and Size Acceptance: A Personal History

*Josephine Cranberry**

Growing up during a time of empowerment of many groups of people, I came to a time when I finally felt freed of that last boundary for me, size. This is my personal recollection of how the political movements from the 1950s through the 1980s led to my acceptance of my size and appearance and my subsequent involvement in the size acceptance movement. The issues of integration, the red revolution, the women's movement, gay rights, and war and peace were all going through changes during my adolescent and young adult years. They were about accepting people as people and that no one is superior to anyone else. I liked those ideas. I believed in them. This is my path and my perceptions of the changes that were occurring.

I come from a small town in northern Minnesota. My first recollection of a human rights issue occurred when a woman in our area was elected to Congress. Her name was Coya Knutson. She was a member of the Democratic Farmer Labor Party. Because she had a unique set of qualifications due to her involvement in her father's business and a connection she could make with the farmers, she had gotten the vote. However the party was reluctant to support her. Although there is some debate over the motivation, a campaign to remove her from Congress was launched in her husband's name. It was called "Coya, Come Home."[1]

My young sense of righteousness caused me to become quite enraged that her husband would think he had a right to demand she come home and leave her job in Congress. I was not aware of the political machinations that caused the campaign, but I did see the message that a woman should not be in Congress. It was 1958. I was 13. At that time feminists were certainly around

---

*Josephine Cranberry, a nom de plume to protect my privacy

but not as vocal in the media as they later became.[2] Nonetheless, I had a strong belief that, as a woman, I ought to be able to have whatever profession I wanted. It just did not seem right to me that I needed to choose between being the perfect woman as portrayed in the media or a woman with a career. The *Feminine Mystique* by Betty Friedan was not published until 1963, but in it she described the schizophrenic split women of the '50s faced between playing the traditional role of wife and mother and being educated for something else.[3]

I was in high school in the late '50s and early '60s. The civil rights movement for racial equality was blossoming. I read about it in the newspapers and watched it on television. Integration of the schools was an explosive and compelling situation. We also had magazines like *Time* and *Newsweek*. High school sociology class work was pretty sanitized. We were not yet reading the early books that described the civil rights movements. In seventh grade, we were sneaking, snickering, and sharing pages from *Peyton Place*, which at least unbuttoned sexually repressive ideas.[4] At that time abortion was illegal, and birth control pills were not yet available. We women were just beginning to think about sexual conduct differently.

When I was a senior in high school, we had a social studies project to help sensitize us toward stereotyping. We were asked to answer some questions anonymously. One was, "Would you rent a room in your home to a negro [it was the politically correct term at the time]?" Nearly everyone said "yes." Next question, "Would you rent a room in your home to an Indian [it was the word used at the time]?" Half of my class said "no." In northern Minnesota, there were very, very few black people. Maybe a few were college students or professors at our local state college.

There were enough Native Americans so that non-natives felt threatened and not willing to give up their privilege. We had Native Americans all around us, a silent group of people, living on the edges of town or on reservations. Stereotypes abounded. A few Native American kids attended our high school, but they were not embraced. Although the fight for civil rights for African Americans and Native Americans was not specifically linked in their political actions, I saw them to be the same fight. As a result, I listened and watched what was happening to Native Americans in my community. I did not like it.

My best friend, who was white, was dating a Native American college man, and soon I was dating his best friend, another Native American. I expect that the majority of my community may have been shocked, but my parents took it in their stride, and the boy and I suffered no ill effects from the short-lived romance. I did go to the local reservation for a Pow Wow. My girlfriend and I were among the very few white people there. The drumming was wonderful. I felt a part of the place. I was shocked at the abject poverty and worried about how the children fared in the winter. My concern about civil rights for others was awakening. The American Indian Movement[5] was not formed until 1968, after I graduated from high school and college, but I remember that there was a stirring of activism much earlier. I learned about it from my friend's boyfriend. He was older, far more articulate, and believed in the theory that Native Americans needed to become educated to take their place in American society.

I went to a high school assembly and heard a female war reporter and photographer talk about her work during World War II.[6] I was so impressed; it made me feel, that I, as a woman, could be a reporter. Hence, when I enrolled at the University of Minnesota, I majored in journalism. I felt I had made the choice to attend college and become a career woman in a nontraditional field because I just did not fit the image of the traditional woman. I was not thin, and I wanted to get out of my small hometown and to be more than a wife, who would cook, clean, have babies, and do her husband's bidding.

The story of my personal battle with size acceptance goes back to my childhood. I was a skinny kid. I wanted to be bigger. In sixth grade I was 4'11" and weighed 89 pounds. I was never any good at athletics and was picked last for teams. I thought it was because I was too skinny. However, athletics for girls were not considered to be important. I happily attended a country elementary school, and I truly enjoyed competing to be the smartest kid in the class. Everything changed when I hit puberty, gained weight with a mature body, and started junior high school. No longer part of a small country school that was very homogenous, I was now attending junior high in town where I was exposed to the issues of economic strata, status, and personal image. I fell from the comfort of the economic norm to being a poor chubby kid who was not in the popular clique. My body matured quickly, and I perceived myself as too fat. I immediately started dieting. I thought I would never be able to join the popular kids' group, and thus gain personal happiness and fulfillment, because I was fat. I wanted to be pretty, popular, and have a cute boyfriend. Who didn't? Losing weight seemed to be the answer. Then I could deal with being a female and find ways to leave the mean streets of my hometown.

We may not have had the social media of today, but we had *Seventeen* and *Glamour* magazines and they were filled with diets and turning oneself into a female image of someone's imagination. At 5'3" I thought I ought to weigh 103 pounds, like Sandra Dee. I weighed about 125 pounds. Thus began the perpetual diet to lose 20 pounds, and, as the years progressed, I lost and gained much more.

Having lived through this dichotomy of images of believing that equal rights applied to everyone, that we all had a right to do what we want, look the way we are, and yet knowing that I was not seeking a path consistent with the female role I was supposed to live, I knew something was wrong. I was not familiar with the struggles of the earlier feminists and did not have access to the stirring of a reenergizing of the movement. The idea that my physical form was no one's business but mine was not in my mind.

In 1963 I started college. There was so much promise: Black people and Native Americans were winning legal battles for equal rights,[7] and everyone was rejecting the middle-class value of being rich and privileged. No one wore cashmere sweater sets and pleated wool skirts as the rich girls had worn in high school. Everyone wore cutoffs and sweatshirts, and even I could afford that kind of clothing. We were excited about having a new president (John F. Kennedy) who was Catholic and supportive of our progressive beliefs. Personally, I was excited about being out of my small town and living away from the obligations of family that included being the oldest, caring for my sisters, doing housework, and working in the family fishing bait business. So, even though I was fat and female, I was still pretty darn happy. Then the bottom fell out of my world. Shots were fired in Dallas, and we wondered if the promises of our youth had been cut short. JFK was assassinated. We grew up.

In college, the issues of the day were segregation and race and ethnic rights and then the Vietnam War peace movement. Since I grew up in northern Minnesota, I had no personal experience of what segregation and racial bigotry had done to black people. But I could certainly see that it was wrong. There were not too many people around me who adopted the position that segregation was a good idea. I read the *Fire Next Time* by James Baldwin[8] and took a sociology course called "Race and Nationality in the United States." My childhood friend had married her Native American boyfriend, and they kept me apprised of the growing "Red Movement." I really wanted to join the Freedom Riders[9] who were registering black people in the South, but I could not financially afford to stop working to do so. I was attending college on a shoestring and a prayer. The most I could do was wear a black armband and picket the auditorium when George Wallace[10] came to speak. I attended pro–civil rights and antiwar rallies. I was so outraged that discrimination occurred because of the way people looked. It felt like the world was with me in that opinion, but then my world was a large liberal university.

For my first two years of college, I dated, but I had expected to have a career and not get married. However, I had a chance to let go of my revolutionary ways and get married. Despite my size, I had dated and met a boy who reluctantly decided to marry me. I adjusted my goals, felt more normal to accept the role I was expected to have, and got married. I met my husband in the dorm cafeteria where I worked, and two years later we got married right out of college. Although he accepted my fat body, he expected it to get smaller. After we got married, he went into the Air Force and I got a job teaching elementary school. In my generation, the boys all had to deal with the draft, so they got an exemption, enlisted, or left. My husband went through Reserve Officers Training Corps (ROTC) to avoid the infantry in Vietnam, and so he was obligated to four years as an officer in the Air Force. I was against the war and the military. I felt I had to make up for the fact that

I was a liberal, fat, and had a job by being a super homemaker. I scrubbed and cleaned the house, learned how to cook, did all the household shopping, paid the bills, and put on parties for his crew. During that time I got fatter, and he harassed me about that. I blew up to a size 14. I joined Weight Watchers and lost 30 pounds. I'm a lifetime member.

I was still trying to be a good wife. It was kind of rough to be a military wife, and a peacenik, but I had always not fit in. I dieted, losing, gaining, more dieting. As much as I felt like a rebel of sorts, it never dawned on me that I was very much conforming to size expectations.

Toward the end of my marriage, after my husband got out of the military and we had moved to San Diego, I recall an incident that demonstrates his attitude about my size. We went to the movies with my best friend and her husband. She was passing me a box of popcorn, and my husband knocked it out of my hand so I could not eat it. She mentioned it later and I realized that I had not noticed. I guess I thought I deserved it.

The beginning of the women's liberation movement, part 2, began while I was married.[11] I started reading Ms. magazine[12] and other books and publications. It was becoming apparent to me that I definitely had a right to an equal partnership in my marriage, and I did not have one. While he was in Vietnam, I experienced for my first time as an adult, not a college student, that I could make my own choices. It felt good. I had a great time. When he returned from Vietnam, I spent a year trying to find a way to integrate my newly found freedom with our marriage, but it just did not work. He still picked on me about my size, and I was still dieting and he was adamant that he make the decisions on how the money was to be spent. He was begrudgingly doing the dishes and helping with the laundry.

Our marriage ended in 1973 when I walked out. In 1974, Congress passed the Equal Credit Act,[13] which prohibited discrimination in consumer credit practices, in part, due to gender. Turns out, I probably did not have a leg to stand on when I insisted that our community property should be equally divided.

The following year I took an extension class about the feminist movement. It was taught by a small, dark-haired professor who told us that her 30th birthday goal was to lose enough weight to fit into a pair of leather pants. I had not yet been introduced to the concept of size acceptance, but, somehow, this felt wrong. Here we were, studying about women's rights, the unfairness of the objectification of female images, and dumping expectations of living in traditional women's roles. The goal of the leather pants? It was not consistent with the other revelations.

The class was enjoyable. It is difficult to explain how it was in 1975. I had seen us go through issues of segregation and the Vietnam War. We had eschewed middle-class life, and we had moved on to a vastly more free attitude toward enjoying sex and drugs. We were talking about women not being required to be a wife and mother, but being able to work in professions that had been dominated by men, and about not dressing as expected. We talked about these issues and then expanded the ideas to our own personal lives. We talked about our own career objectives, the relationships that we wanted to have, not liking to cook and clean and do traditional women's tasks. We got out mirrors, flashlights, and speculums and took control of our own female parts.

I joined the National Organization for Women.[14] And, I began to read the books. I read *Sisterhood Is Powerful*[15] and the *Female Eunuch*.[16] Germaine Greer articulated the relationship between the feminist movement and the objectification of a woman's body. Though I did not notice at the time, she clearly stated, "Whenever we treat women's bodies as aesthetic bodies without function we deform them and their owners."

To me, feminism meant an opportunity to be me with no expectations that I fulfill a traditional female role or look a certain way. How women dressed and wore their hair and makeup was evolving. They stopped wearing dresses. Pants for women had been around for a long time, but we had been expected to wear them only for casual occasions. Pants were prohibited in the workplace and church. When I started college, we still wore dresses, gloves, and hats if we went downtown to shop. I had to put on a dress to work in the dorm cafeteria. I wore pants as a teacher only starting in 1970, and then only pantsuits were permitted. We stopped wearing makeup and shaving our underarms and legs. We no longer ratted (teased, back combed) or used tons of hairspray on our hair as we had done in the '50s and '60s. We did not burn our bras, but we did stop wearing them.

My roommate and I attended this class together. We bought bib overalls, got contraceptives (the Pill was now available outside of marriage),[17] and brainstormed about careers. I was working for the welfare department, and I commented that I saw our appeals unit doing legal analysis and I thought it was interesting. My roommate and I looked at each other, and I said, "I ought to be a legal secretary." We both did a double-take and said in unison, "Legal secretary, hell no, I ought to be a lawyer!" That is how I decided to attend law school.

My roommate was also recently divorced and went on to locate a suitable husband and have a fairly traditional life, but she has always been a free spirit underneath it all, and I would like to think that our early days have inspired her to openly accept and enjoy her children's life choices. Feminism meant freedom. It also meant personal acceptance, and that really had to do with body image.

There were also issues of personal health and care. *Our Bodies, Ourselves*[18] instructed us that we could participate in the health and care of our bodies.

It taught respect for our own bodies. There was at least one book that made no specific judgment on size, *The Well Body Book*.[19] Although it did discuss nutrition, there were no specific comments on weight loss. It did have a message about paying attention to one's body and respecting it. One of the main concepts is the "3 million-year-old healer" because the body has had 3 million years of evolution to reach this point in time. The concept is to live life in concert with one's body's needs. Although my notes from 1974 in this workbook reflect my concern over minor body ailments, I did not relate the concept of the book to size acceptance.

It had begun to puzzle me as to why women in the movements were still fussing about their size. Feminists had adamantly refused to be sex objects. They wanted to be equal partners. However, when I attended a National Organization for Women meeting, for example, I felt like a lesser woman because I was fat. I saw no fat pride. It almost seemed like I still had to be superwoman: brighter, more athletic, and thinner to prove that we women were not only equals but superior to men.

In 1980 I joined the California Feminist Federal Credit Union founded in 1975.[20] The manager was fat and a lesbian. We became good friends, and she introduced me to the idea that it was okay not to diet. She was comfortable in her body and saw that being concerned about size was another issue of objectification of the body. From my volunteer work with the credit union, I became involved in other feminist groups and became somewhat acquainted with gay rights. It was important to me not only as another civil rights issue but because I had a close family member who was gay. These civil rights issues were moving from the political to the personal. Later that year I invited a fat lesbian coworker to be my roommate. She ushered me into her office and quietly asked if I knew about her lifestyle. She moved in, and we had many long conversations about size and gay rights, and we learned from each other.

The first time I saw fat addressed from a feminist viewpoint was in a book called *Fat Is a Feminist Issue*,[21] which I read in about 1982 when I was 37. The book pointed out that a woman's disdain of her body was rooted in antiwomen feelings all around her. The objectification of a woman's body engendered feelings of inadequacy if she did not meet the expectations. Unable to meet the expectations of the "perfect" body, she regressed to only the nurturing of food. It was self-hate that reverberated like a boomerang. The book did have a message that if one only felt okay about her body and let go of certain attitudes about food, lesser eating would seep in, and, voilà, weight loss.

All of the logic of why I "overate" still did not explain why diets did not work for me. I still felt somewhat like a failed human being, albeit, an enlightened feminist one. I suppose I thought that if I just believed my body was okay, as only a feminist could believe, I would lose the weight and live happily ever after. I tried free eating, and, no, I did not lose weight. However, I was beginning to be freed from the concept of dieting, and I was beginning to feel that anyone who was critical of my size was doing so from a bigoted viewpoint.

It took a few more years, one last diet, graduating from law school, and finding a permanent job before I finally moved into a belief that I was a totally acceptable human being, fat and all. I decided that it was magic thinking that if I only believed I had an attractive body, I would have one.

In about 1986 I became personally involved in the size acceptance movement. At that time, there was no Internet, no e-mail, no Facebook or other social media. There was the telephone, television, newspapers, books, and person-to-person contact. It was personal contact that got me involved. Next door to the nail salon I patronized was a small, independently owned dress shop for fat women. Regretfully, today the independent brick-and-mortar dress shops no longer exist. But they did at that time. When I got my nails done, I usually checked in with the owner about her latest fashions. Eventually, we chatted about the size acceptance movement.

She was a size acceptance advocate and used her shop as a springboard for that advocacy. She kept flyers on hand for fat dating services and social groups and other fat-friendly businesses. She held workshops on the issues that fat women face. She had fashion shows. She networked with other size-friendly organizations. There was another fat-size dress shop that I visited. She too had fashion shows and other events. This included a fat belly dance duo performance. I later learned they were the originators of the Fatimas, a fat belly dance troupe that still exists today and that I later joined. I then learned that one of those women, along with a couple of other partners, had another group that not only had a dating service but also hosted house parties and dances. It was called Mor2Luv. I signed up for the dating service and ended up talking to the maven of matchmaking who was also one of the most knowledgeable people I have met.

Then I went to a Mor2Luv house party and experienced that tremendous relief to be among strangers that might not judge me by my size. Having observed the journey of human rights movements, I knew this was the right next step for me.

Once I became involved in Mor2Luv, I became more politically involved in the size acceptance movement by participating in informational booths, pickets, and workshops. In the late 1980s in Southern California, there was a community of size acceptance groups. They were social and political. I loved being back in the mix. It felt similar to my contact with the civil rights issues previously noted above. I joined the National Association for the Advancement of Fat Acceptance (NAAFA).[22] I went to size acceptance dances and met more wonderful people. I developed enduring friendships with women at group events sponsored by NAAFA chapters and also by Mor2Luv. I found clothing vendors that designed clothing just for me. It was a beautifully diverse crowd. Many shared my passion for supporting the civil rights movements that I had seen as I was growing up.

I spent time with a bunch of fat folks and those who support and love them, and I certainly loved and respected them, and I came to the conclusion that I could love and respect myself. How could I look at myself and view me as ugly or unacceptable? They were not ugly or unacceptable. Because I had watched and been immersed in the civil rights movement, it was an easy progression to see that fat people ought to be respected and treated equally too.

In the end, I would say that civil rights and the belief that one is entitled to those rights is a very personal process. We need the political clout to address the issues. However, first we must truly believe we have the rights.

My involvement in the size acceptance movement has helped me address the issues I now have as a very large woman. Today I am a retired judge who is 350 pounds with a 22-year-long relationship with a man of color. This life is a result of my personal evolution and choices given to me by the battles that people have fought for all of our civil rights. Peace and love.

NOTES

1. Minnesota History Museum, Coya Knutson, http://www.mnhs.org/library/tips/history__topics/119coya_knutson.html, citing research and writings by Gretchen Urnes Beito and other secondary and primary sources, June 30, 2013.

2. Alice S. Rossi, ed., "Feminism and Intellectual Complexity," in *The Feminist Papers* (New York: Columbia University Press, 1973), 615.

3. Betty Friedan, *The Feminine Mystique* (1963; reprint, New York: Dell, 1970), 11–12.

4. Grace Metalious, *Peyton Place* (New York: Messner, 1956).

5. Laura Waterman Wittstock and Elaine J. Salinas, "A Brief History of the American Indian Movement," accessed June 23, 2013, http://www.aimovement.org/ggc/history.html.

6. John Simpkin, "Dickey Chapelle," September 1997, http://www.spartacus.schoolnet.co.uk/JFKchapelle.htm#source.

7. Susan Cianci Salvatori, project manager, National Historic Landmarks Program, National Parks Service, U.S. Department of Interior, "The Civil Rights Framework Study," 2002, revised 2008.

8. James Baldwin, *The Fire Next Time* (New York: Dial Press, 1963).

9. Cicely Morris, director, Congress of Racial Equality (CORE) publications, "Freedom Summer," accessed July 7, 2013, http://core-online.org/history/freedom_summer.htm. During the summer of 1964 white college students from the North were recruited to assist in voter registration in the South. They faced threats, harassment, and more. Their participation to end voter suppression of African Americans in the South brought attention to the inequities, though there was resentment that the struggle had been going a long time, and only when the whites got involved did the inequities gain national attention.

10. Richard Pearson, "Former Ala. Gov. George C. Wallace Dies," *Washington Post*, September 14, 1998. Wallace's notoriety came from his staunch resistance to integration of schools when he was governor of Alabama. He promised to stand in the schoolhouse door. He backed down when President Kennedy sent in national troops. In 1964 he ran for several Democratic primaries and found some support in the northern states. Later in life he renounced his anti-integration position.

11. Rossi, "Feminism and Intellectual Complexity ," 629. The author delineates the feminist movements into three periods with some breaks in between when those generations personalized the issues into their own lives. The first peaked in the 1850s, the second ran from 1900 to 1920, and the third began in the late 1960s.

12. Jone Johnson Lewis, *Ms.* magazine, July 8, 2013, http://womenshistory.about.com/cs/periodicals/p/p_ms_magazine.htm. *Ms.* magazine was first published in 1971 as a feminist publication. At the time of publication, there was controversy over the sexism of titles for men and women. Men had the marital status-neutral "Mr." but women had only a title of "Miss or Mrs.," which did designate marital status. Feminists chose a marital-neutral title of Ms.

13. Equal Credit Opportunity for Consumers, 15 U.S.C. section 1691(a) provides that "it shall be unlawful for any creditor to discriminate against any applicant, with respect to any aspect of a credit transaction—(a) on the basis of race, color, religion, national origin, sex or marital status, or age." California Family Code Section 1100 provides that either spouse has control of community property as of January 1, 1975. Before that it was the man who had control.

14. History of the National Organization for Women at http://www.now.org.history/, July 2006. The National Organization for Women was founded in 1966 by Betty Friedan and Dr. Pauli Murray after a battle with the Equal Employment Opportunity Commission over providing a provision about sex discrimination in employment for the implementation of Title VII of the Civil Rights Act of 1964.

15. Robin Morgan, ed., *Sisterhood Is Powerful: An Anthology of Writings from the Women's Liberation Movement*, 1st ed. (New York: Random House, 1970), xiv. The editor collected articles from different types of women's viewpoints in an effort to demonstrate many issues involving discrimination against women. She distinguished the women's movement from other civil rights organizations as the "male-dominated counterfeit left."

16. Germaine Greer, *The Female Eunuch*, Bantam paperback ed. (New York: McGraw-Hill, 1970), 29.

17. Chana Gazit, "The Pill," a film transcript at http://www.pbs.org/wgbh/amex/pill.pill.html/. The birth control pill was first approved by the Food and Drug Administration in 1960, but there was great controversy over its use. Several states made it illegal to use it. For states who allowed its sale, the policy during the 1960s was that it would be distributed only to married women. It was credited as beginning the sexual revolution, enabling women to do actual family planning and have careers. It was also beginning a time that allowed greater sexual freedom.

18. Boston Women's Health Collective, *Our Bodies, Ourselves: A Book by and for Women* (New York: Simon and Schuster, 1973).

19. Mike Samuels and Hal Bennett, *The Well Body Book* (New York: Random House, 1973).

20. http://www.Credit unionaccess.com/cui21917.htm. The California Feminist Federal Credit Union was founded in 1975. It merged with another women's credit union in 2009, and that credit union was liquidated October 12, 2012.

21. Susie Orbach, *Fat Is a Feminist Issue* (Paddington Press, 1978, New York and London).

22. http://www.naafaonline.com.dev2/about/index.html, website for NAAFA. NAAFA was founded in 1969. It describes its mission as a "civil rights organization dedicated to protecting the rights and improving the quality of life for fat people. NAAFA works to eliminate discrimination based on body size and provide fat people with the tools for self-empowerment through advocacy, public education, and support." Through the years the organization has changed, but in the 1980s it was an activist group with social and political activities.

4

Resisting Negative Stereotypes of Female Fatness

Lori Don Levan

Fatness is one human condition for which people (at least in the United States and many Westernized cultures) can be openly ridiculed and discriminated against because it is perceived as a "condition" that can and should be changed. This "condition" crosses race, ethnic, gender, sexual orientation, and economic borders, so that the damage that is done by persistent fat phobia and bigotry has the potential to affect everyone. In general, fat phobia acts as a policing agent that controls all people through relentless regulation of the body. Specifically, fat phobia acts as a policing agent for women that serves to subordinate their place of power within a patriarchal context. In this chapter I will discuss how fat women are constructed through the visual image, one example through advertising and the other through artistic practice. While both may seem to have similarities, it is through their differences that I hope to construct a path for resistance to negative stereotypes.

In the February 2000 issue of *Talk* magazine, Bijan Fragrances ran a three-part series of advertisements that had been turned down by every major fashion magazine on the market. Tina Brown, then editor of the magazine (and a good friend of Bijan's), loved the advertisements and ran them without question. In the meantime, all other magazines that had willingly run his ads in the past (*Vogue* and *Town and Country*, to name just two) refused to run this particular series without explanation. It was only after Tina Brown accepted the advertisements for *Talk* that the magazines that had initially refused to take them had a change of heart. Not happy with the response and change of heart, Bijan decided to allow the advertisements to run only in *Departures*, *Vanity Fair*, and *Esquire*. The question for Bijan became why such a fuss?

This series of advertisements was generated by a company that was no stranger to outrageous advertising, yet had been embraced in the past in spite of any controversy. Bo Derek was once featured with diamonds in her hair and partially nude along with Bijan and his young son (clothed). In another ad campaign, Bijan featured a young woman in Muslim dress holding a bottle of Bijan perfume with the caption "Jammal, you might as well know the truth … I'm in love with Bijan." Why were these new advertisements rejected? Could it have been that the advertisements featured, quite predominantly, the nude image of a very fat woman, the model named Bella? The advertisements were designed to mimic the style of several artists (Botero, Matisse, and Rubens) and featured Bella wearing nothing but a very tiny set of heels along with Bijan himself as the "artist" portraying different roles in the three scenarios (titled "Bella," "Motel," and "Siesta").

Presented with a sense of humor, the images appeared to be beautifully constructed photographs of Bella and Bijan in the artist's studio and the boudoir. Bijan was broadly smiling in two of the images. Assumptions that the images were digitally assembled and that there was a very low probability that Bijan and Bella were ever in the same room together when the photographs were taken were part of viewer criticism of the advertisements. Cynthia Miller, Bijan's art director at the time, said in an interview with the author that the advertisements were indeed actual photographs.[1] Although she insisted that the images were not retouched any more than what would be done for Cindy Crawford (a popular model at the time), Bella's body surface in the images appeared to be flawless. These images were featured on Bijan's website where one could answer the question "What do you think of Bella?"

WHO IS BIJAN?

The concept for the Bella ads came from Bijan's need to create a work of art.[2] He wanted to use the images of Rubens, Matisse, and Botero as the inspiration. He felt the colors and treatment of surfaces along with the celebration of the voluptuous female body would be a wonderful counterpoint to the elusive experience of the actual fragrance that was being advertised. In particular, Bijan wanted to use photographs in order to re-present the images of Botero that he admired. Bijan was in full control of the design of the advertisements and considered himself to be an artist in the process. Bijan may have considered himself to be an artist, but he was first and foremost a very smart businessman. A designer of men's clothing, jewelry, and fragrances, he also designed fabulous showrooms in Beverly Hills and New York to showcase his work. He used Michael Jordan and various other celebrities of that time to promote his name and developed a website to promote his merchandise.

After the advertisements appeared, Bijan made some appearances on television, including *The Roseanne Show* along with Bella on March, 29, 2000.[3] His discussion of the Bella advertisements included much attention to the fact that he wanted to create great art. Bella supported his effort and seemed to be honored by the fact that he had chosen her for his subject. Bijan stated that he based his decision to use Bella on the fact that she radiated a kind of inner beauty that supported her external beauty. Bella was very comfortable with the nudity and stated that she loved the idea "that he had created a master-piece, as if it were anybody else, and it's something that could be shown in a museum, that I could be hanging in a museum."[4] Bijan referenced Matisse, Rubens, Monet, and Botero with the emphasis of the discussion on the accepted belief (at least in the art world) that all of these artists created great works of art that featured nude fat women. He stated, "To me, every woman is beautiful."[5] He acknowledged that he was known for creating controversial advertisements and that Bella was an example of something unusual that he could not understand was being rejected. He emphasized the nudity that existed in any major museum was perfectly acceptable and known by his major clients. The rejection that he experienced was unexpected based on what he thought he knew about his clients and what he assumed they would tolerate. He discussed his feelings. Why wouldn't the magazines carry the advertise-ments? Could it have been the nudity? Cynthia Miller and Bijan himself never really received any explanations; just a flat "no" came from publications that regularly ran pictures of nude and seminude women and had run his ads in the past. What was making them so uncomfortable? Could the "controversy" really have been a "tempest in a teapot" self-generated to bring attention to the advertisements of his new product?

Bijan was very happy that so many people supported the advertisements once they were published. He had with him a huge stack of e-mail that he supposedly received within the two days before the interview. Unfortunately, he was unable to read any of them on the air. Cynthia Miller in her interview reported that 95 percent of the responses were positive and the rest were of no consequence since they were in such a minority. Following is one of the responses:

> Bella is enchanting . . . when I was a child I saw beauty in everyone I met—some of the most beautiful people I met as a child were elderly, fat, retarded, deaf . . . I can remember trying to squint my eyes to get wrinkles because of one particular elderly lady I admired because of her lines which drew a picture for me on her face. I think it is about time artists were allowed to express beauty with diversity. Ever since I was old enough to read—I became disillusioned with advertisements in their [narrow-minded eyes' view] of what is considered beautiful—cosmetically altered young girls—a vision that no woman on the street could ever accomplish—and women have come to view themselves as ugly, fat and have lost their beauty because the image given was impossible to live up

to. I give Bijan applause for taking a "risk" in his advertisements. I would like to see more diversity in advertisements—especially where women are concerned.[6]

Discussions about these advertisements with different people revealed a concern and disbelief over the shape of Bella's backside. Heated discussions over whether or not the photograph was altered because "nobody's butt could possibly be that shape, it is too perfect!" caused me to consider the question "Who is Bella?" Not much was said about the context of the advertisements, the reference to art, whether or not they were beautiful, or even if the people who looked at them had an opinion about whether or not they liked them. "Beautiful Bella" was also described as having vibrant blue eyes, tiny hands and feet, and a bubbly personality, and her weight distribution was characterized as being bottom and extremity heavy. Because of this fragmentation, part of what became important to this story was Bella's voice. She was represented in various places but never actually contacted. She was mentioned in several newspaper articles pertaining to the controversy over the ad campaign; however, most of the attention in those forums was placed on her actual weight in pounds. This was also the case on *The Roseanne Show* where she was discussed as the 400-pound model that Bijan used for his advertisements. Bella's presence on the program was diminished once Bijan entered the stage. The few comments that she did make were masked by Bijan's presence. Bella's identity as a person was also masked since she had no role to play other than the object/subject of Bijan's efforts.

Previously, Bella was featured on the cover (and in the feature article) in the February 1998 issue of *Dimensions* magazine (a magazine for BBWs [big beautiful women] and the men who love them). She also had some experience making erotic videos. One of her videos, titled *Bella-Dancing*, produced by Sandy Sabo at Russo Productions, begins with Bella in a natural park setting seductively eating a banana. She is reclining on the ground, and when she finishes, she gets up and walks over to a small tree. As she passes behind the tree, she magically transforms into an exotic dancer in full belly dancing regalia. Persian music is playing and she proceeds to dance for her imaginary audience. This scene is followed by her in the pool swimming and finally in the boudoir modeling sexy lingerie. The video ends with her taking a bubble bath. The images are fairly tasteful although Bella herself occasionally appears to be awkward and very self-conscious.

These are the forms of representation in which Bella was found; however, her voice was never present. In each case she was constructed as a mute object of desire. Bella's power was dissipated through the examination of her parts. The supposed controversy over the advertisements also seemed to be fragmented, and my research most often led to Bijan's website and several newspaper articles that were all worded as if they were being taken from the same press release. The "controversy" characterized above seemed to be self-contained along with Bella's silence.

Resistance against fat oppression is an unusual concept for many people to grasp. In some ways, people might think that fat prejudice is not really prejudice at all. Fatness is just something to be concerned about, especially since "obesity" has become a supposedly national "epidemic."[7] Speaking about hunger, Naomi Wolf argues:

> Female fat is the subject of public passion, and women feel guilty about female fat, because we implicitly recognize that under the myth, women's bodies are not our own but society's, and that thinness is not a private aesthetic, but hunger a social concession exacted by the community. A cultural fixation on female thinness is not an obsession about female beauty but an obsession about female obedience.[8]

She goes on to say:

> Fat is portrayed in the literature of the myth as expendable female filth; virtually cancerous matter, an inert or treacherous infiltration into the body of nauseating bulk waste. The demonic characterizations of a simple body substance do not arise from its physical properties but from old-fashioned misogyny, for above all fat is female; it is the medium and regulator of female sexual characteristics.[9]

In this context, the image of a powerful fat woman is threatening and has to be disempowered. Bella is voiceless and her mute participation in the act of creating an advertising image keeps her powerful large body in check. Bijan's diminutive stature is counteracted by his placement in the images. He is the powerful artist in charge and she is his mute muse.

If fatness can be imagined as an "obesity epidemic," obsessive behavior against it can be justified. If we speak about "it" in metaphoric terms, then we can detach ourselves from it and keep it at arm's length where the fat person stays as the faceless other that exists in the margins. Bella's back was turned to the viewer in the images and her face was visible only in a slight profile. This otherness is continually represented in the media whenever a story on some sort of obesity research/weight loss miracle is being reported. How often are the images of fat people walking the streets shown where only their fat torsos are visible? Barry Glassner in his book *The Culture of Fear* argues:

> Not only do we use metaphors to help us understand fatal illnesses that most of us are poorly equipped to comprehend scientifically, we also create certain illnesses, what I call "metaphoric illnesses," to help us come

to terms with features of our society that we are unprepared to confront directly.[10]

I argue that "obesity" is one of the metaphoric illnesses that Glassner speaks of. Keeping women internally focused on the most difficult thing to control about their bodies distracts them from the power that they stand to gain in the external world. But, what of the woman who refuses to submit? What happens to her in the process? How can she resist?

Michel Foucault argues that bodies are produced through disciplinary practice. In Foucault's chapter "Docile Bodies" from *Discipline and Punish*, he describes his theory of the disciplined body using the example of the soldier for which every aspect of his life is controlled—from dress, spatial experiences, and activity as it relates to a complex system of power relations.[11] While Foucault's arguments center mainly on the male body, Sandra Bartky argues that there are three categories of disciplinary practice that produce feminine bodies: "those that aim to produce a body of a certain size and general configuration; those that bring forth from this body a specific repertoire of gestures, postures, movements; and those that are directed toward the display of this body as an ornamented surface."[12] She describes feminine disciplinary practice as it relates to diet and exercise, grooming, and spatial activity. "Woman's space is not a field in which her bodily intentionality can be freely realized but an enclosure in which she feels herself positioned and by which she is confined."[13] Fat women take up space in very undisciplined ways according to this scenario where nonconforming body size is a constant reminder of failure in the disciplines that create femininity.

Susan Bordo argues that feminist writing on the body helped to move critical thought from the metaphor of the "body politic" (coming from Plato and Aristotle) to a new metaphor of "the politics of the body."[14] Drawing on Michel Foucault's theories, Bordo describes how modern power operates in this arena. Power is a

> dynamic or network of non-centralized forces ... that these forces are not random or haphazard, but configure to assume particular historical forms ... [and] prevailing forms of selfhood and subjectivity are maintained not through physical restraint and coercion, but through individual self-surveillance and self-correction to norms.[15]

Referring to the panoptic nature of power that Foucault discusses in *Discipline and Punish*, her assessment of feminist writing on modern power relations and the body allows for the possibility that "cultural resistance is ubiquitous and perpetual."[16] She proposes that feminist discourse has moved beyond dichotomous thinking about social control to "acknowledging that creative and resistant responses [can] continually change and disrupt it."[17] Creative agency, therefore, allows "for the eruption of 'difference', and even the most subordinated subjects are therefore continually confronted with opportunities for resistance, for making meanings that 'oppose or evade the dominant ideology'. "[18]

Fat phobia is positively reinforced in our society because internalized oppression allows for open criticism of the fat individual as well as that individual's capitulation to that criticism. Creative agency, however, is what allows fat women who are critical of this type of oppression to move from a marginalized position in ways that are beneficial to them. Oppositional discourse creates resistance to the power relations that maintain current beauty ideals for all women. It is through this discourse that the invisible hand from the margins can reach out to inscribe its mark on the ideology of the mainstream. While it may cause a rift initially, the action of resistance is absorbed and alters the mainstream in subtle ways as long as it is persistent.

Elizabeth Young-Bruehl describes prejudice as a silencing agent that takes on various forms. Prejudice through categorization can be rejected through the "territory of definition" where resistance is used to dismantle the "oppressive categories."[19] In contrast, she describes obsessional prejudices in a more complex manner. They have "in their operating modes ways for suppressing their victim's insights into the nature of their victimization, as well as suppressing their victim's resistances."[20]

Bell hooks uses the term "sites of resistance" to describe the location of resistance to oppression. In her essay *In Our Glory: Photography and Black Life*, she discusses the importance of photography to black communities in the segregated South where making and displaying photographic images was an important activity that afforded black individuals the ability to represent themselves according to lived experience. For hooks, "The walls of images in Southern black homes were sites of resistance."[21] The photographic image in this context would be considered visual resistance to negative stereotypes of the black body.

> All colonized and subjugated people who, by way of resistance, create an oppositional subculture within the framework of domination recognize that the field of representation (how we see ourselves, how others see us) is a site of ongoing struggle.[22]

She saw the camera as a political instrument used to "resist misrepresentation as well as a means by which alternative images could be produced."[23] While hooks's arguments are used to frame discussions on racism, they are useful when describing representation and fatness.

Hooks also uses the term "gestures of resistance" when describing challenges to authority and says that there is "power in looking."[24] According to hooks, Foucault allows for the possibility of resistance in a power system of dominance where

> Even in the worst circumstances of domination, the ability to manipu-
> late one's gaze in the face of structures of domination that would contain
> it opens up the possibility of agency . . . he invites the critical thinker to
> search those margins, gaps, and locations on and through the body
> where agency can be found.[25]

Resistance is the action that individuals or groups of individuals take against prevailing ideology, and sites of resistance are the physical manifestations of that resistance. Sites of resistance are essentially visual in that they rely on visual cues to transfer their ideologic challenge. Persistent resistance brings about change. For example, even though fat phobia is so deeply rooted in our society, there are fat activists who regularly protest discrimination through their actions.

Laurie Toby Edison is a West Coast artist and activist based in San Francisco, California. Originally a metal artist and jeweler, she became a fat activist out of a need to effect change. Her first photographic body of work, *Women En Large: Images of Fat Nudes*, became a self-published book in 1994.[26] The black-and-white images included nudes of women in familiar settings like their homes, gardens, and on the beach. This body of work has been embraced by the feminist community in Japan and has been shown extensively there. Her collaborator, Debbie Notkin, provided the written text for the book and has participated with Edison as copresenter in many conferences, activist events, and exhibitions of the work. From Edison's website:

> Photography carries with it a profound sense of reality. We are flooded
> with a constant barrage of images from advertising and media, using beauty
> and gender to persuade, to sell, to influence. Laurie Toby Edison's nude
> photographs subvert this reality. Her beautiful fat nudes . . . are powerful
> counters to this flood of commoditization. Edison believes that what you
> are forced to see every day constrains how you look at the rest of what
> you see. Her work demonstrates that art can counter those constraints by
> providing fresh, uncontestable, uncommercialized images.
>
> If we can imagine a body image that is individual and not determined
> by anyone's distant gaze, that relies on difference rather than sameness,
> and that is sensual as well as visual, the entire universe of discourse
> shifts. In the wake of the shift, everyone has the right to determine her
> or his own level of visibility and only his or her own, no one else's.
>
> Edison's work encourages both the people being photographed and
> the people who look at the photographs to define their own visibility,
> and expand their vision of beauty.[27]

The disruptive nature of fat activism is in its visibility. Through persistent resistance to negative stereotypes of fatness, alternative images of beauty, corporeal experiences of fatness, and critical questions concerning marginalization can be asked and presented through the construction of sites of resistance. Kathleen LeBesco argues, "In terms of identity, the lived experience of fatness inhabits the same space as, and yet diverges from, other influential subject-marking experiences, such as the embodiment of race and sexuality."[28] Relying heavily on the theories of Judith Butler and Elizabeth Grosz, LeBesco makes a claim for "queering fat bodies" in the sense that difference in relation to fatness can be politicized if we consider the corporeal aspects of living in fat bodies as they relate to theories of difference. "Queer activists and theorists propose forms of political action that recognize individuals both as subjects with the capacity to act and as subjected to larger forces over which they have less control."[29]

Controlling discourse through agency in the formation of sites of resistance allows a space for new ideas to be debated without necessarily compromising the uniqueness of the marginalized person and her or his lived experiences. Therefore normalization, moving from the margins to the center, does not necessarily have to happen in order for sites of resistance to be effective. LeBesco argues that "identities are never merely descriptive; rather, they are strategically performed."[30] In this sense "communication as political practice" becomes part of the process of constructing sites of resistance where an "anti-essentialist" point of view allows "the ability of human actors to participate in the creation of meaning."[31] The communicative nature of and creative agency involved in creating sites of resistance make them effective tools for change where the fat body does not have to be compromised in order to conform to any type of beauty ideals other than the ones that are determined by the agents in charge of the sites.

Edison's images are constructed through collaboration with the subjects where they have agency over the outcomes of the photographic act. Her creative process relies on her subject's participation. In their keynote address to the conference Fat Attitudes: An Exploration of an American Subculture and the Representation of the Female Body,[32] Laurie Toby Edison and Debbie Notkin talked about their need to promote change through their work. They argued that a fat woman "always carries both those labels with her; she is always fat and always a woman."[33] Their presentation was accompanied by slide images from Women En Large: Images of Fat Nudes, and the debate that they encouraged set the tone for the rest of the conference. While their message was multilayered, they expressed a need to break away from dichotomous thinking about fat female bodies. Notkin stated:

Early in our work together, long before Laurie started taking photographs, we learned that the statement "fat women are beautiful" does not simply stand in radical opposition to the belief that fat is ugly. If we say "fat women are beautiful" without caution and qualification, many people hear us say "thin women are ugly," or at the very least, "if fat women are beautiful, then thin women can no longer be beautiful." This is not our message; in fact, it speaks to the tendency of our culture to demand simple dichotomies (if one thing is good, the opposite must be bad). This also speaks to the ways that people (and women in particular) have been taught to fix on anything which might undermine their self-esteem . . . We had to extend our initial statement, "fat women are beautiful," to the even more radical "beauty is abundant and available to all."

Edison and Notkin discussed the images from *Women En Large*, connecting them to issues concerning beauty, health, race and ethnicity, aging, sexuality, disability, gender identification, and oppression as they related to the fat woman. The visual images that Edison created were not separate from her activism. Talking about them and exhibiting them was a political act that speaks to her (as well as Notkin's) need to communicate ideas to as many people as they could reach and it still has relevance today. They also spoke of the educational aspects of their activism. Two examples were cited: one of the experience of an anorexic woman who was asked to write an essay for the book and the other of the experience of showing the work to young school-aged children in Japan. Both of these experiences showcased the ways in which the work was used to educate and to encourage critical self-reflection.

Notkin spoke of her experience as one of Edison's models and she noted that aside from the personal liberation that she experienced, "the aesthetic quality of Laurie's photographs, her trained and intuitive understanding of composition, light and shadow, form and balance, is the reason that they are so powerful as a tool of social change." Edison and Notkin ended their presentation saying, "Each fat woman who asserts her right to live fully is a harbinger of the world we all want to live in. Each ally who supports us is a bulwark of the effort."

Laurie Toby Edison played an important role in leading me to be a fat activist. As she and Debbie Notkin continue to advance their cause both here in the United States and in Japan, I realize that what they leave behind is the need to effect change. They inspire in their work in both word and deed as well as through the visual images left behind as a reminder, a call to action. I am hopeful that this work and work by others will help to expose the internalized oppression we all carry within us. I was able to recognize the internalized oppression I carried because of their work. This "awakening" helped me to become an activist and work toward social change and educational reform. It is from the margins that radical ideas will come. It is through resistance that change will happen.

NOTES

1. Personal phone interview with Cynthia Miller conducted in October 2000.

2. Any references to Bijan and the actual construct of the Bella advertisements are taken from the interview mentioned above.

3. Video copies of the broadcast and transcripts were provided through Burrelle's Information Services via the Internet in October 2000. Any quotes from *The Roseanne Show* were obtained through these sources.

4. Excerpt from *The Roseanne Show* transcript, March 29, 2000.

5. Ibid.

6. This quote was taken from examples of e-mails given to the author by Cynthia Miller after the above-mentioned interview.

7. Especially since the U.S. Centers for Disease Control has made it a top priority.

8. Naomi Wolf, *The Beauty Myth: How Images of Beauty Are Used against Women* (New York: Anchor Books, 1991), 187.

9. Ibid., 192.

10. Barry Glassner, *The Culture of Fear: Why Americans Are Afraid of the Wrong Things* (New York: Basic Books, 1999), 153.

11. Michel Foucault, *Discipline and Punish: The Birth of the Prison* (New York: Vintage Books, 1977).

12. Sandra Lee Bartkey, "Foucault, Femininity, and the Modernization of Patriarchal Power," in *The Politics of Women's Bodies: Sexuality, Appearance, and Behavior*, ed. Rose Weitz (Oxford: Oxford Press, 1998), 27.

13. Ibid., 30.

14. Taken from a chapter in *Feminist Theory and the Body: A Reader*, where Bordo is excerpted from *Unbearable Weight* and various lectures.

15. Susan Bordo, "Feminism, Foucault and the Politics of the Body," in *Feminist Theory and the Body: A Reader*, ed. Janet Price and Margrit Shildrick (New York: Routledge, 1999), 253.

16. Ibid., 254.

17. Ibid.

18. Ibid., 255.

19. Elisabeth Young-Bruehl, *The Anatomy of Prejudices* (Cambridge, MA: Harvard University Press, 1996), 458.

20. Ibid., 459.

21. bell hooks, *Art on My Mind: Visual Politics* (New York: The New Press, 1995), 59.

22. Ibid., 57.

23. Ibid., 60.

24. bell hooks, *Reel to Real: Race, Sex, and Class at the Movies* (New York: Routledge, 1996), 197.

25. Ibid.,198.

26. Laurie Toby Edison and Debbie Notkin, *Women En Large: Images of Fat Nudes* (San Francisco: Books in Focus, 1994).

27. Accessed August 10, 2004, http://www.candydarling.com/lte/. Her current website is http://www.laurietobyedison.com/index.asp, accessed June 5, 2013.

28. Kathleen LeBesco, "Queering Fat Bodies/Politics," in *Bodies Out of Bounds: Fatness and Transgression*, ed. Jana Evans Braziel and Kathleen LeBesco (Berkeley: University of California Press, 2001), 80.

29. Ibid., 81.

30. Ibid., 83.

31. Ibid., 84.

32. Held at Teachers College, Columbia University, February 27–29, 2004, and organized by the author.

33. Quoted from the keynote address to the Fat Attitudes conference, February 28, 2004.

5

Anatomy of an Activism Campaign: A 2003 Action against Weight Loss Surgery Marketing

Marilyn Wann

In late August 2003, I organized an action to respond to a particularly hateful example of weight loss surgery marketing, a print ad in the *San Jose Mercury News* that longtime fat activist and Health at Every Size expert Deb Burgard, PhD, had noticed. Compiled here are reports from participants, from both the time of the action and their recollections now, a decade later, as well as an excerpt from *Los Angeles Times* coverage of the action.

There are several goals involved when I speak out against weight loss surgery. Whatever the setting, I hope to

- Challenge stereotypes about fat people.
- Share information about the long-term complications and dangers of these surgeries.
- Raise awareness about Health at Every Size alternative as a viable way for people of all sizes to seek health and happiness.
- Protect people of all sizes from being pressured or frightened or manipulated or coerced or blackmailed into agreeing to weight loss surgeries.
- Criticize uncomplicated promises about improved health.
- Criticize postsurgical promises unrelated to health, such as relief from weight discrimination in the workplace or other kinds of negative treatment.
- Reaffirm people's total right to bodily autonomy.
- Make clear that, whatever people may or may not intend, opting to have weight loss surgery by its very nature reinforces a weight-based definition of health, of mobility, and often also of what an enjoyable or worthwhile life is—and these definitions perpetuate anti-fat attitudes.

- Expand availability of weight-neutral and fat-positive options, both in health care and in all aspects of life.

These hopes seem just as uphill to me now in 2013 as they did in 2003, perhaps more so. They also seem like minimum requirements for a society in which people of all sizes can live well.

From a *Los Angeles Times* article, "Fat, and Happy about It; Despite the health risks of obesity, activists demonstrate against weight-loss surgery, which they say is dangerous, demeaning," from February 19, 2004, written by Lisa Richardson:

> The newspaper ad inviting fat people to learn about El Camino Hospital's new weight-loss surgery program held out the opportunity to be not just a thinner person, but a better one.
>
> "It's not what you have to lose," the Mountain View, Calif., hospital ad said. "It's what you have to gain. Pride. Dignity. And Better Health."
>
> Marilyn Wann, 5-feet-5, 270 pounds and darn proud of it, scanned the ad and fumed: How dare they imply that fat people are not proud, or that dignity is reserved for the thin? Wann threw down the newspaper. Then she smiled and began to e-mail her friends.
>
> At the hospital's weight-loss surgery workshop in October, Wann and a handful of others blended into the crowd, most of them at least 100 pounds heavier than doctors say they should be. They listened to the surgeons—then Wann blew a whistle.
>
> The infiltrators jumped up, whipped off their clothes and, clad only in bathing suits (Wann in a pink two-piece), danced through the stunned audience with the words "Fat+Pride" and "Fat+Dignity" marked on their stomachs.[1]

* * *

From Marilyn Wann . . .
[Posted to the Show Me the Data e-mail list on August 29, 2003]
Hello:
Last night, a group of merrymakers and rabble rousers of all sizes—calling themselves the Bypass-the-Bypass Brigade, or BBB—disrupted the sales pitch of some weight-loss surgeons.

Inspired by the surgeons' own advertising strategy . . . —photo of a lovely fat woman in swimsuit, standing proudly on diving boar—text that said, "It's not just about what you lose. It's about what you have to gain. Dignity. Pride. And better health. With our surgical weight loss program, you stand to gain a lot. And the leaders in the field of obesity surgery are ready to help you."

. . . The Bypass-the-Bypass Brigade attended the surgeons' sales meeting, waited stoically until the presentation was done, then disrobed to reveal their flabulous, swimsuit-clad selves (both one- and two-piece). They wore belly signs that depicted happy, bouncy stomachs and the word, "Dignified!" or "Proud!" or "Healthy!" They also chanted this slogan gleefully as they danced about the room, smiling at the fat people in attendance and handing them sassy hot pink handouts.

At one point, the evident ringleader of the BBB (in hot pink bikini) exclaimed, "When someone comes at you with a knife to cut off vital organs, the smart thing to do is run far away from the scary person . . . so that's what I'll do!" (She glanced mock-fearfully at the surgeons, then grabbed up her gear and danced out of the meeting room.)

Evidently, after the BBB action exited the sales meeting, conversation continued, with many fat people among the audience voicing strong challenges to the surgeons' claims. [NOTE: See follow-up post, below, for description of the Q&A team.]

One fat woman asked, "What data do you have that fat people who undergo weight-loss surgery live longer than fat people who don't undergo the surgery?" The surgeon assured the crowd that such data exist, although she was unable to offer any specific journal cite. The questioner said she had searched the literature herself and found nothing on the topic. When pressed, the surgeon offered to take the questioner's e-mail address and respond privately.

A young fat man was heard to say, "I want to thank you for this presentation, which so horrified me that I will never consider having this surgery." Several audience members made pitying noises at him, and a representative of the surgical team (was it the bariatric nurse or the nutritionist?) said, "Why, are you scared???" He said, "No, I'm not scared. I just would never risk my health in this manner." The surgical proponent pushed him, demanding, "Have you actually researched this surgery?" To which he responded, "Yes, I've researched the surgery, including the three friends of mine I've watched die from it." The woman said, "I'm sorry," as she walked quickly away.

Earlier, this same young man had asked the surgeon why he couldn't have dignity and pride right now, without having his stomach cut off. The surgeon said she didn't intend for people to be offended by the ad, but that it was meant to show how dignified and proud her "obese" patients are already, but especially so when they make a choice to "move forward" for their health. She then made the unsupported claim that there was no one in the room who was free of health problems.

The Exhibit A fellow (who has lost 234 pounds since Surgeon-Girl cut off his stomach 14 months ago), suspiciously had no saggy skin and no "before" photo of himself to offer. However, his story rang true to knowledgeable types in the crowd, because he exhibited all the signs of exercise compulsion, anorexia, bulimic thinking, and Stockholm Syndrome. Judging from his story, he also seemed to have no life interests aside from his very physical job and his food regimen.

The organizer of this action would like to express that she has never experienced (in her rather adventurous life to date) such heart-knocking, fear-defying, full-body exhileration as she felt last night. She is convinced that more such festivities will occur at surgical sales meetings around the San Francisco Bay Area . . .

Wheee! – Marilyn Wann, FAT!SO? chick

PS: Heartfelt thanks and humble awe for the bravery of Connie, David, Greta, Hadas, Jeff, Laura, Shirley, Susan, Yalith (and Natalie). And *especially* to Deb Burgard for alerting fat community about the hospital's advertisement and for coming up with the brilliant phrase, "bypass the bypass."

* * *

From Marilyn Wann:
[Posted to the Show Me the Data e-mail list on September 2, 2003]
Hi, lists:
I just want to make a clarification to my giddy posting of last week, the one about an action at a weight-loss surgery sales meeting.

I was writing in a mock-clandestine style, and so failed to explain that there were actually two teams of rabble rousers involved in the action. One team wore swimsuits and made merry. The other team attended the meeting, sat through the swimsuit team's pranks, then asked challenging questions of the surgeons. I reported the Q&A team's actions in my earlier message, without making that clear.

I'm worried that what to me was a coy stylistic choice may have led some readers to imagine that the swimsuit team's action inspired immediate skepticism on the part of attendees who were actually considering the surgery. That wasn't the case. Although I do fervently hope our combined actions caused some people to rethink their options. . .

Sorry for any confusion! – Marilyn Wann, FAT!SO? chick

* * *

From RGA in May, 2013 . . .

I was assigned to be a question person and handed a yellow legal pad. I was among a dozen or so eager fat activists, headed for a South Bay hospital to protest the new, so-called "roux-en-y" gastric weight-loss surgery, for which there was a presentation by a leading surgeon.

Half of us were planted as the Q&A people, and the other half were dressed in gloriously bright muumuus, posing as actually interested fat people. I remember it being difficult sitting through that presentation and keeping a serious face on, all the while pretending to be interested in what the surgeon was babbling about. At one point I caught the eye of the doctor, and may have flashed a look of pure derision in reaction to the disgusting procedure he was touting as the newest way to good health. [The lap-band surgeon.] Was he French? Did he have a thin, blonde assistant with him? Did they mean for the name [Roux-en-Y gastric bypass] to come from a delicious thickener made of butter and flour? Was I on a weird reality game show? These details are murky. What has stayed with me, though, are the looks on the faces of fat people listening to him, hanging on his every word, looking for salvation—desperate for the answer to the "dreadful" state of their body, and their constant companion: Shame.

Eventually, the Q&A started; I don't recall the questions I or others asked. At that point, I could barely hold it together anyhow, knowing what was about to happen. All of a sudden, a whistle blew (Marilyn), and the muumuu folks stood up, yanked off their coverings to reveal bikinis and fat-positive words written all over their exposed flesh. All of them started to yell and chant at the dumbfounded, ashen-faced presenter: "Fat is beautiful!" and "Fat is healthy!" and other taboo and barely-spoken phrases, while telling the attendees they didn't have to buy into this. They then ran out of the room.

I got to stay in my seat, feigning shock. The best part of this: witnessing the surgeon and his assistant become pale and speechless. The worst part: seeing the heartbreaking reaction of other fat women who were attendees remark how rude and obnoxious those people were, "when I'm just trying to do something healthy for myself!" It was a powerful event for me, as it put those words of body-positivity out there into normal-land (and I can only hope at least one woman heard and adopted these words), yet it also illuminated the fact that most fat people blindly put faith in doctors—if they tell these women that putting a rubber band around their stomachs is healthy, and that their post-surgery digestive problems are UNrelated, they WILL believe it.

I came out of that action with a roller coaster of emotions, running from exhilaration to doom. My activism since then has been in smaller ways, like when I had a massage client the other day, who was a fat woman talking about only if she could lose 10 to 25 pounds, she would be . . . I responded with a suggestion of letting go of the numbers weight game, and instead concentrating on moving about more and getting more active, despite what number she weighs; it tends to distract people from actually using their bodies, and to increase shame. She thought about it and said, "Maybe I was right about that!" Small victories . . .

* * *

From NB, PhD, in May, 2013 . . .
Looking back on my field notes from the 2003 action I noticed that one of the first things I wrote down was the copy from the print advertisement that had inspired the action. It read:
"It's not about what you lose. It's about what you have to gain. Dignity. Pride. And better health."
I can honestly say that attending that meeting and being a tangential part of the courageous action that took place that night did indeed solidify the dignity I felt in my own body. It left me with a renewed sense of fat pride and community, and I have no doubt that questioning the messages of the surgeons that night and to this day has improved my mental and physical health.
At the time I was a little conflicted about my role in the action. On the one hand, I wanted to be a part of the brave group of swimsuit-clad fat activists jumping up and declaring our wholeness and humanity. After all, at the time I was a Padded Lily [a synchronized swimming team made up of fat women] and no stranger to public bikini wearing, even as I had never so directly confronted those wishing to surgically alter my perfectly wonderful fat body. On the other hand, I was researching my dissertation on the "obesity epidemic" and the sociologist in me wanted to be able to step back and chronicle the action and to be able to stay in the room and see how the surgery peddlers responded to being so viscerally called out on their fat hate and profit motives. As much as I wanted to be counted among the brave and fabulous fatties that intervened that night, I am glad I was there to see what happened after they left.
In spite of the surgeons' and event organizers' best efforts to pass the action off as the theatrical efforts of a bunch of crazy fat women in denial about the catastrophic health consequences of their "morbid obesity," the feeling of the room had changed and the feeling of enthusiasm on

the part of those seeking information on weight loss surgery was forever lost. For the rest of the evening there was a palpable tension in the room and the questions asked by potential patients were more critical than they had been earlier in the session. Since 2003 I have continued to research weight loss surgeries for my dissertation and later for my recently published book, *Killer Fat*. In the course of this research I have attended dozens of surgery information groups and surgery support groups. I attended a weekend-long weight loss surgery convention and I have interviewed many post-operative bariatric surgery patients. In immersing myself in the world of weight loss surgeries I have never seen the tone of a support group or informational session change as quickly as it did that evening in 2003. I have never seen such critical questions asked at a pro-surgery event and I have never seen the standard surgical line of fat=death and surgery= rebirth so powerfully subverted by the presence of whole, beautiful, power- ful, fat bodies the way it was that night. I know lives were saved that night. I know that like me, people are healthier for having attended and more whole for having been in that room and witnessing that action, and not for the reasons the surgeons had hoped.

* * *

From DB, PhD, in May, 2013 . . .

I think I might have seen the ad in the paper of a nice-looking plump woman in a swimsuit on a diving board and the text said something about, "Don't you wish you felt more pride?" or some BS thing and I may have called you, enraged,—I do remember brainstorming with you about calling the action, "Bypass the Bypass," and you called Connie and they did some videoing at the event (I was not there).

* * *

From YF in May, 2013 . . .

I remember I wore a hot pink bathing suit. My adrenaline was pumping as I tried to reassure myself it was okay to be disruptive in the interest of get- ting out information about fat acceptance that isn't widely disseminated. I think we danced around a bit and handed out our fliers. The seminar attendees looked confused more than anything else. I don't think they quite understood it was a political action because they didn't know yet why weight loss surgery would be a political issue. Hopefully, they read our fliers and found out. We all went out for Chinese food afterward. It was fun.

* * *

From HRW in May, 2013 . . .

I remember having fun, for one thing. In no particular order, I remember there being at least one person there, who was considering the surgery, who was disturbed by us, and that pained me more than anything. The hilarity of the doctors, especially one, their faces, that's invigorating. I love having fun when I'm doing this kind of stuff, otherwise it's just too morose and demoralizing. We're up against huge power.

This goes across any political focus issue. The most effective message or signage is something that has humor. I've always loved standing there with the signs that said, "Eat me!"

Two people attending the meeting, Samoan or Tongan, they were very disturbed. I just don't know a way to do something that is both disturbing to people who need to be disturbed and supporting the people who we need support. I don't know if we can do that at the same time. To make potential allies not alienated from us. How do we support people who we think we know better than, or at least I do.

i knew someone who had the surgery and it didn't work. They gained back every last ounce and were then dealing with serious depression around the issue. The person's parent—I don't know what to call it: stupidity, or what adjective — encouraged another sibling to do it, with clear proof that for at least one of her children it did not work. The assumption was that it's better to die trying, even if you knew it's not going to work . . . the extent to which families can pressure somebody.

The surgeon who was the main presenter was a young woman with brown hair who was very perky and pretty glib. She definitely had a PR thing going, completely without depth. Trying to get people who hadn't decided about it and their families. If i remember correctly, there were probably about 20 to 25 people, including family members, not just the patients. That plays a huge factor, the thinking of the family: "If you only did this, I wouldn't have to worry about you any more."

I remember the comment of somebody who was with us, David, just so clearly because of the way it upset the surgeon. David sat smack in the middle of the whole thing. By that point, the surgeon already knew I was trouble or anyone she deemed to be associated with us. She took a question from him. He said he wanted to thank her because before the session he'd actually been thinking about or considering the surgery, and this information session permanently scared the hell out of him from ever doing it. The surgeon, who was the main presenter, said, "Oh really, why?" She was not sure that he was with us or not. She wanted to improve her presentation. He wouldn't give it to her. At the end, it was still unclear who he was and that destabilized the whole meeting.

Except for disturbing people who were considering doing it because they thought that was their best option, I thought that was perfect.

As to my own contributions, I was in a suit to embody some kind of legitimacy, or five minutes of she's-not-with-them time. I'm not sure that worked.

It's still a complicated issue.

I know someone who looks me in the face and explains to me why she did it. I can't exactly judge her. It's a horrible thing, especially in most every other person I've talked to or heard of. But I still don't feel like I can sit in judgment of people who do it. I don't really want to do that. I remember feeling at that time very much more righteous about it. Anybody who did this obviously didn't love their body and if they didn't love theirs, then they didn't love mine. It has nothing to do with me from their perspective. That rejection is actually not the full picture. If we're to take into consideration, we need to talk to people who've actually done it. Maybe I would be less judgmental of their choice and focus more on what the bigger culprit is. Because I feel like I put too much responsibility on the person who's electing to do that. Whether it's just mental or condescending or some other adjective that's not flattering. That's my personal thing to work out.

The bigger culprit is why they're pushing people who weigh 200 pounds to do it. Why they're not publishing what the real picture is like before, during, and after. I still don't think we have good data. I don't think that even if it was collected and shared it could be had, because it's still a relatively new surgery. It's being touted as the antidote to everything including even if your pantyhose run. If I thought this was the answer to my own health concerns, I wouldn't want to be judged. I have not been convinced that it's that kind of answer and I haven't seen enough data based on what they came in with and what they came out with.

I don't know if what we did changed what the surgeons do for the ultimate benefit of everybody. I don't know if what we asked about the data really spurred them to look at it. [Hadas asked, during the meeting, for data on death rates.] I wonder if we keep doing this kind of thing what effect it would have. If we did it again, I would ask more questions than point fingers. I would ask the kind of questions that demonstrated support for the people who were there, in some way.

Susan, my ex, she had all the information that could be had. She was brilliant. I don't know whether any way that anybody treated her around her decision would have changed her mind. I would ask questions that showed consideration for people who were terrified and considering it.

* * *

From SS in May, 2013 . . .

I've told this story to people time and again, so yes, I do remember something about that action.

We had seen print advertisements which, as I recall, depicted a "fat" (actually fattish) woman on a diving board and had some comment or other about how she'd feel ever so much more comfy out in the world in her swimsuit if she'd just lose weight—preferably by having weight-loss surgery.

This was particularly insulting/annoying to those of us fatties who swim whenever and wherever we please, and aren't particularly troubled by hating our bods—in fact, I, for one, am an adherent of the biblical saying: "Be kind to your ass, for it bears you." (At least I'm TOLD that's biblical, but I can't cite chapter and verse.)

ANYWAY, we went to an orientation (read: sales) meeting at the hospital to hear all the glorious things weight-loss surgery could do for us. As usual, we were the fattest prospects in the room. We wore swimsuits with dresses over them. Some of us had size-positive messages painted on our bodies. We watched the film (or was it a slide show?), passed around a piece of the gear that's used in the operation (lap band was it? I just know we considered stealing it to keep it as a souvenir), and upon an appointed signal, we stood up, stripped off our dresses and proudly displayed our fat, swimsuit-clad, message-painted bodies, and disrupted the meeting.

I hear that after that meeting, they didn't do open orientation meetings ever again, and one had to register and be screened to attend.

* * *

From CS, August 30, 2003

Hi all:

I sure did try to get it on video, but the experience was so intense that I mistakenly pushed the stop button just as the event started. Major bummer! What I did get is an amazing interview with Marilyn right after we infiltrated the meeting, and she rocks! The emotion is all there. She was then joined by the rest of the brave people who were part of the protest, and the conversation is great. I am truly sad that my pounding heart caused me to make a blunder, but 'C'est la vie.' I've signed on for the future protests. It was unbelievable.

A comment from a former bulimic about the poster child held up by the weight loss surgeons—the man has an eating disorder. It was frightening to hear him speak and especially scary to see that he was the one the surgeons were holding up as the success story. He had eating disorder written all over him. Wonder how long he'll be alive. And, as the major point made by the surgeons was that they are increasing the longevity of their patients, I'd love to check in with this man in 10-20 years. Scariest comment of his that evening—"I do eat chicken now, but it has to be really soft, because if not, it comes right back up. But the good thing is that since I have no acid in my stomach, it comes up tasting just the same!"

I also observed that the woman sitting right in front of me was probably their 6 week patient who was going to be available for questions after the presentation. The entire time the surgeons were talking about the procedure, she was nodding profusely. The frightening part was when the surgeon talked about "dumping," when a patient eats sugar in any form and it immediately causes diarrhea and vomiting. The woman's head bobbed up and down and she had a pathetic smile on her face. I really wanted to tap her shoulder and ask her if she was enjoying life.

Another sad part of the presentation was that the people who are unsuccessful in losing weight after the surgery were described as not able to change their lifestyles to include exercise and healthy eating habits. First of all, how can anyone have healthy eating habits when their stomach can only hold 2 oz. of food? And can only have 2 tbsp. of water at one time? Obsession in the making, naturally. I kept thinking how great it would be if the surgeons would save their patients' money by helping create environments for people of all sizes to move without fear of harassment, and real education about healthy lifestyles. At $35,000 a pop, just one surgery payment (as Marilyn said) could create a gym for fat people at the hospital.

I went from the meeting to my friend's house and we watched the video footage with three girls—ages 10, 12 and 14. Their comments, along with my friend (who has lived in Australia for the past 10 years and is blown away by the American sickness of obsession with thinness) were that they wished they had been there to participate in the protest, and that they want to be present at the next one. I explained the surgeons' presentation and all were disgusted, appalled, ready to take action. So—on to the next demonstration. This time I'll watch for that little red "rec" button on my screen!

Marilyn, you rock!
Your sister in the revolution,
Connie

* * *

From CS in May, 2013

The experience I had at the demonstration stays with me to this day. I have not let go of the sadness I felt for the man who stood up to talk about his "success," the man who was severely suffering with an eating disorder. I think one of the things that stands out most is that he was no longer able to exercise. There are so many things wrong with that! Not just that he can't truly be healthy without movement, but that the pleasure and joy that come with movement were taken away from him by the surgeons who profited from his unhappiness with his body. Over the years, I've heard many sad stories about people who have elected to have the surgery, and each time my heart breaks a little bit more. Yet with that heartbreak I become more dedicated to The Body Positive's work to support people in living in, loving, and caring for the bodies they inherited from their ancestors. The powerful memory of Marilyn and the others who participated in the demonstration in 2003 stays with me always and helps to fuel my passion for transforming the beliefs about beauty, healthy, and identity that cause body hatred. Though I bungled the job of documenting the event, the experience was recorded in my brain and will remain there for the rest of my days.

NOTE

1. Lisa Richardson, "Fat and Happy about It," *Los Angeles Times*, accessed January 5, 2014, http://articles.latimes.com/2004/feb/19/local/me-fat19.

6

My Fat Body: An Axis for Research

Rebecca D. Harris

To label someone obese obscures that person; all that can be seen is the fat. They become stigmatized and this anthologizing process turns them into a mere object. Obscure Objects of Obesity, an interdisciplinary MA project, explored, through my arts practice, the discursive notions of the fat body as a deviant body, a body that needs to be controlled, restricted, and recontoured to reach "satisfactory" normativity. The project developed from the emphasized awareness of my body, prompted by anticipating the gastric bypass I was due to have in August 2012. However, this was with trepidation, as initially I was ignoring this stigmatized subject matter only to discover unintentional explorations discernible in the artworks I was creating at the time. Despite my unease of placing myself in a vulnerable position, I decided to "come out" as a fat woman and originally set out to create a project responding to the psychosocial and physiological changes brought on by the weight loss surgery. It transpired, though, that the concerns with the "normalizing" extremes I was about to put myself through led me to discover counterdiscourse of the fat female body, and I felt a reconciliation with my fat identity so, at short notice, I canceled my operation.

Despite not having the surgical procedure, I continued with my inquiry. The project situated my fat body as an axis for research, as my experiences of being a fat woman and related investigations of obesity were at the core. Although instigated by personal events, the artworks have much more social relevance. For autobiography, from the ancient Greek *autos* ("self"), *bios* ("life"), and *graphy* ("writing"), is a retroactivity using hindsight in which an individual communicates a significant period in their life.[1] Such an approach conveys something of the individual, and I wanted my story to impact on wider social discourse and debate. Therefore I chose autoethnography, from the ancient Greek *autos* ("self"), *ethno* ("culture"), and *graphy* ("writing"), a combination of autobiography and ethnography, which "seeks to describe and systematically analyze personal experience in order to understand cultural experience."[2] Autoethnography enabled me to utilize my own experiences to discover and comment on matters much beyond my personal self. The art-works do not didactically address the theme of obesity; they are much more subtle, creating an alternative paradigm of the subject matter. Furthermore, viewers can bring in their own narratives, bodies, and experiences to read these autonomous artworks.

In losing my house I explored the theme of Home, in losing my mother I explored the theme of Death, but when I was about to have a weight loss operation, in which I would lose a significant and life-changing amount of weight, I chose to ignore this subject matter. Reference to the body is a thread that ran throughout these prior themes, in particular the skin in the Home project, and the body became more explicit in the recent project Fetish. Preceding Obscure Objects of Obesity, and following the theme of Home, Fetish explored gender divisions within the home, investigating the material-ity and object-hood of domestic and do-it-yourself paraphernalia into object-based sculptures. During the development of this work, and despite no intentionality, weight loss surgery worries manifested within these artworks. It was not necessarily what is to be read by the audience, but was what I saw reflected in the artworks, which was the basic apprehension of alien interven-tions of my body and the subsequent sagging skin. Despite the lack of attention to a theme so pertinent in my life, I realized that the autobiographical tenden-cies, which had previously propelled my inquiries, could be reestablished. The artworks were clearly embodying my concerns and this was an opportunity to fully embrace and explore the subject of obesity emerging from these artworks.

A gastric bypass, which was the procedure I was just weeks away from, during the conclusion of the Fetish work, makes permanent gastrointestinal alterations. It restricts consumption and causes malabsorption through the creation of a small pouch from your stomach and then a shortening of the small intestines. Seeking to normalize my abject body, which I had spent a lifetime disavowing, and despite so much focus on "this" body, I had divorced the physicality or rather the reality of my body with my identity and became a repudiator of my own physical existence. In the book *The Absent Body*, Drew Leder utilizes both medical and phenomenological theory to create the term "dys-appearance" to argue that in day-to-day life the body is self-effacing, at most it is surface body, and through some form of "dys"function it thus "appears."[3] My effacement was extreme; I was ignoring my body, but following the clinical pathologizing process I could no longer ignore myself and thus I profoundly "dys" appeared. Brought to the fore was the heightened sense and awareness of my body's failure. Furthermore, knowledge of the data on mortality rates, surgical complications, impact on quality of life, hair loss, malnutrition, and excess sagging skin, all sought to compound this

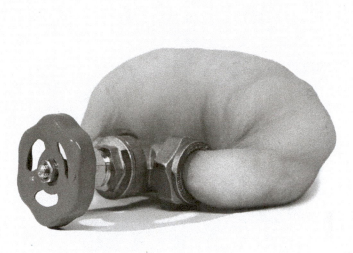

Figure 6.1 Rebecca D. Harris, *Untitled (stop valve)*, 2012. (Courtesy of Rebecca D. Harris)

"dys" appearance. Therefore, considering my previous tendencies to use personal narrative, it became of no surprise how such acute phenomena would affect my practice. Paisley Livingston states, in his book *Art and Intention*, that deeds of intention in art making can occur both consciously and unconsciously, irrespective of whether the artist is aware of their actions.[4] Intention existed, regardless of whether I was consciously aware of it; those Fetish artworks assimilated biological and psychological concerns about the forthcoming surgery. *Untitled (stop valve)* (see Figure 6.1) became emblematic in referencing alien biomechanical alterations of the viscera. A second distinct piece from this previous work, *Life Sucks* (see Figure 6.2), illustrated the simple fear of sagging skin and the loss of female body definitions. Integrated into this project are both the artworks themselves, and their concepts and materials, which were to influence upon subsequent artworks.

Significantly, the fear of creating a body of work on a personal and stigmatized subject matter sheds some light onto my reluctance to address this theme earlier. I was very anxious about making this decision, and despite the self-evidence of my fat body, I saw myself as "coming out" as a fat woman. It was a means of personal acceptance and declaration, which Eve Sedgwick states as "a renegotiation of the representational contract between one's own body and one's world."[5] However, I considered I would not be fat for long, as I would rid myself of my life's stigmatized body and soon be "normalized."

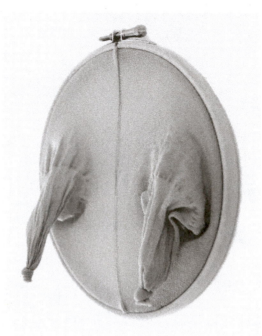

Figure 6.2 Rebecca D. Harris, *Life Sucks*, 2012.
(Courtesy of Rebecca D. Harris)

Australian feminist Samantha Murray considers the experience of the lived fat body as one in suspended animation, waiting to become thin and be accorded personhood while residing in a "constant disavowal of one's own flesh."[6] As I developed my interests in fat studies and activism, I felt a form of reconciliation with my identity as a fat woman and horrified by the extremes I was about to put my body through. Just a few days before I was due to have my surgery I canceled the operation. Although I did not have the procedure, I persisted with my inquiry. Drawing from my embodied experiences, previously mentioned, I remained as an axis for research, but autoethnography was no longer completely relevant on its own, so I adopted a "triangulation" approach, to include autoethnography, "thinking through making," and discourse inquiry, which I discuss below.

Discourse was recognized as always being an active method of inquiry from the onset of the project. This form of exploration was significant as my subject matter is so heavily entrenched with discourse; as Murray suggests, the fat body is "a site where numerous discourses intersect, including those concerning normative feminine beauty and sexuality, health and pathology, morality, anxieties about excess, and the centrality of the individual in the project of self-governance."[7] Being a "chubby" child and "obese" most of my adult life, I was well aware of the negative ways society saw "me" and how this constituted toward how I felt about "me" and my body. Gillian Rose states, "Discourse is a particular knowledge about the world which shapes how the world is understood and how things are done in it."[8] Furthermore, we categorize and interpret "objects," "subjects," and the "world" only through the structures available to us and are often not aware of those formations that make it so difficult to question.[9] Although I knew what my body and personhood meant in society, I did not consider anything counter to this. I was fully involved in this negative discourse by seeking means to normalize my body so I could literally "fit in." At the time of allowing myself to be operated on, I made *Untitled (stop valve)* (see Figure 6.1). Upon reflection, I saw my anxieties of the alien interventions in this artwork. The piece instigated research into weight loss surgeries and social attitudes toward obesity, which led me to hone in on the physical and societal notions of restriction and control. Following this I discovered a counterdiscourse within fat studies and activism; finally becoming empowered and seeing my body as a worthy entity led me to cancel the operation. By "thinking through making," I dynamically took part in discourse; I was discovering, questioning, and resituating my social place and then contributing, through my arts practice, to those reflections to offer the viewer an opportunity to also take part and question their understandings of obesity.

Although the fat body instigated the research, it was also the "thinking through making" approach that opened up a further realm of discovery. For example, *Deep Seated Anxiety* (see Figure 6.3) aims to unite both inside and outside sites of the body, referencing the related surgical procedures of body contouring and liposuction. For this artwork I did not know what I was going to initially make, just that it would be a form and evolve from there. I covered the form in a lightweight calico, pulled the calico tighter and tighter, creating more and more seams, in order to create a sound base for whatever would later cover the soft sculpture. Viewing the tension within those seams, the number of them, and the semitransparency of the fabric halted any further work. Here I had discovered what was registering reconciliation with an excess exterior to a smaller interior form beneath. Thus by "thinking through making," I not only developed an artwork but explored the discourse of reconstructive surgeries following excess skin from dramatic weight loss that may not have occurred exclusive of this working process.

Life Sucks (see Figure 6.2) has signifying content stemming from the objects used as well as what I have "done" to or with them. Initially, feminist ideas may be construed from the knots created within the material that anthropomorphically references sagging breasts, but it is also the tights and embroidery hoops that signify much more. The found objects are "of the world" and retain their "thingness" as I do not attempt to conceal their identity. Sociologist Julia

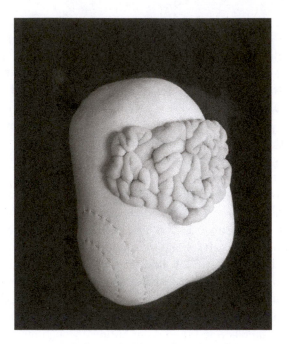

Figure 6.3 Rebecca D. Harris, *Deep Seated Anxiety*, 2013. (Courtesy of Rebecca D. Harris)

Twigg states that in the case of clothing there is a relationship mediated between the body and the social world.[10] She continues, "Forming the vestimentary envelope that contains and makes manifest the body, offering a means whereby it is experienced, presented and given meaning in particular social contexts."[11] Anyone experiencing Western culture would quickly decipher the gender ascribed to tights; from the exposed, yet diaphanously covered legs of women, and the woman's section in a clothing store host a whole range of tights. Emphasizing the surface of her legs, the tights act as a means to conceal her skin, but in turn reveal the intimate contours of her body while acting as a pseudo skin. Although there are tights available in patterned prints and fancy knits like "fishnet," my interests with the materiality of tights is skin mimicry and the potential, of the "oiled" or "sheen" or "nude tights," for body modification. In her cultural analysis of the skin, Claudia Benthien highlights tendencies to fetishize the surface of the female body coming from a focus on the skin being a concealing veil of what makes woman "other," and it is on this surface where that coding of femaleness takes place.[12] Therefore tights became a conduit to explore the discursive contexts of the female skin. Now we move on to a brief discussion of the embroidery hoop. In *The Subversive Stitch*, Rosika Parker discusses embroidery as a subversive feminist trope, used in art as a reaction to the range of discursive formations structured from diverse historical and cultural facets relating to the feminine.[13] *Life Sucks* (see Figure 6.2) does not contain embroidery per se, but the frame references it nonetheless. The functional object tautly holds the fabric for embroidery and is a literal and symbolic "holder" of either a domestic chore or leisurely pastime. Drawing the assemblage of tights and embroidery hoop together, this artwork convenes on the historical, contemporary, and cultural discourse of both woman's work and her body.

In establishing the sites of the biomedical interventions of treating the obese body, the viscera and skin are the two areas I focused on; the skin for its means of communicating the size and history of the body, and the viscera as the locale for weight loss surgeries that then in turn impacts on the skin through the changing body size. In my exploration of the skin as material and conceptual medium, I started with excess skin. *Life Sucks* (see Figure 6.2) uses stretched and unfilled tights to mimetically reference sagging breasts. My preference for tights is reflected in the thoughts of artist Senga Nengudi who selects tights as they relate "to the elasticity of the human body. From tender tight beginnings to sagging . . . The body can only stand so much push and pull until it gives way, never to resume its normal shape."[14] The tights, therefore, not only gave me an opportunity to discuss the inevitable sagging skin of the weight loss surgery patients, but also make anthropomorphic reference to strain upon the body. In my research on the skin, which I later developed as a paper presentation, I retained an autoethnographical approach, and as I was no longer going to have the operation and so retain my inflated skin, I therefore placed my focus on its current stretched state.

In weight gain, arguably no other organ is more physically altered and visually modified than the skin. Flesh, viscera, and bones reside relatively undisturbed as the mass of the body grows around. As the fat swells, the skin expands, transmuting the body toward the discursive fat person. Murray suggests that there are collective negative tendencies to judge the fat body. She states:

> As members of Western society, we presume we know the histories of all fat bodies, particularly those of women. . . . We read a fat body on the street, and believe we "know" its "truth" . . . The fat subject is lazy, not willing to commit to change or to the dictates of healthy living. They are compulsive eaters, they are hyper-emotional; in short the fat body is discursively constructed as a failed body project.[15]

The social gaze is primarily constructed from our experiences with other people. Jean-Paul Sartre observed that one comes to the realization of one's self not just as a being-for-itself but as a being-as-object and being-for-others upon the encounter of the social gaze.[16] Feminine bodily aesthetics, Murray argues, are formed by the relative worthiness or unworthiness bestowed by the heterosexual male gaze.[17] Within the media, men's bodies are "premised on the privileging of masculine bodily strength, power and ability to protect ... whereas the woman's motivations are centered on their appearance."[18] Linking fat as feminine, Murray posits that fatness for men is a feminizing characteristic seen to weaken them, and for women their relationship with fat is a process of obtaining, or retaining, the "normal" body to be aesthetically beautiful or desirable to men.[19] Shifting these notions to the surface, Benthien states that the male body is, historically and culturally, the paradigmatic body, characterized by powerful muscles and veins beneath his skin.[20] The female body retains her "otherness" as what lies beneath her skin is taboo, her body must be contained, and the "skin is a concealing veil."[21] Benthien explains that "undressing a woman of her skin would fundamentally destroy the myth of her being other" and therefore she becomes defined by being both a container and surface with "coding of femaleness [taking] place on the skin."[22] Through my arts practice, I developed a series of machine-embroidered textile pieces that explored the idea of skin as repository; questioning the skin as a container of meaning that embodies femaleness, fatness, and the body's history.

Flaying the skin, its topography became my visual and conceptual medium, so the obvious material of choice, for me, was fabric. Skin and cloth are analogous for their capacity to conceal, and act as a surface, and textiles have a familiar presence throughout our lives and are often referred to as our second skins. It became apparent that I could exploit these notions and not draw just on clichéd analogies, but rather on our intimate relationships with this ubiquitous material. Textiles are much more than an obvious choice, owing to our knowledge of them through touch and proximity to the skin; it was the suitable and fitting choice. In honing my selection I gave preference to working with calico, an unbleached woven cotton in a loom state, and in fact this cheap and insipid fabric is not generally used for any bodily adornment; rather, owing to its primal state, it too is naked.

In this investigation of the fat skin's materiality, I witnessed the stretch mark as something that acts as memorial. They are unapologetic and do not forget a body in excess to become the indices to what the skin endeavors, or endeavored, to contain. The antithesis to the controlled nature of the thin person and the materiality of their body, the stretch marks symbolically render upon the surface of the fat person, a body that is out of control and in strained containment. Benthien states, "The skin is conceptualized as something that is worn, an inescapable garment,"[23] and thus the mass of a fat body is seeking to break its boundaries by displaying the ruptures within its sheathing membrane. Although the male skin can stretch in the same way, Benthien situates the female skin as a locale for female coding, which explains the attitude of feminine beauty being skin deep. In the article "Tracing the Skin's Surface," Melanie Hurst argues that male tendencies to fetishize female body parts lead to beauty endowed upon the surface, and "a superficial ruse or a lure is deeply embedded in sexist contempt for femininity and this contributes to the feminization of the skin."[24] On the veneer of the female body, beauty is interrupted by stretch marks; their emergence is unwanted, which leads to a demand for cosmetic prevention and treatments to a predominantly female clientele. Furthermore, stretch marks have connotations of femaleness in their indexical traces of pregnancies and alongside notions of women aspiring to be stretch mark free, leads to femaleness and stretch marks being inextricably linked.

Upon the calico surface, I sought to elevate the status of the cloth and embellish its surface with what would normally be considered blemishes. The use of embroidery, mostly defined as a feminine craft, became a means to subvert the blemishes and create a seductive surface that abstracted the pattern of the disembodied stretch marks. Using a silky thread, the machine-embroidered zigzag stitches alluded to the materiality of the shimmering stretch mark, in which horizontal tension is created on the top layer of skin when the middle part vertically splits to reveal the deeper layers. This act of destruction and modification in the skin is something also mirrored in the process of embroidery, as Pajackowska argues that "the stitch pierces, punctuates, penetrates . . . and in a single gesture it combines both aspects of the paradox of destruction and creation."[25] These notions can be applied to how the body is modified through cosmetic surgeries in which the hand enacts a power over the material of the body to cut and sew in a reconstruction toward an aesthetic preference.

Penetrating the border, I sought to investigate the areas of the body so heavily associated with the biomedical notions of weight gain and weight loss—the stomach and the intestines. Emerging from *Untitled (stop valve)* (see Figure 6.1), this series of amalgamated do-it-yourself paraphernalia and stuffed tights explore the body's biomechanical state; an object to be dissected, explored, cut, and rerouted as a means to an end, that end being the normative body. Criticized by sociologist Bill Hughes, biomedicine, the approach of modern medicine, has limitations in its consideration that "health is solely dependent on its repair [and] ignores the thinking, feeling and social aspects of healthy human existence."[26] Hughes goes on to state a preference for biopsychosocial medicine as "human existence is, simultaneously, biological, psychological and social."[27] This is in fact a term I found to fit my own approach to the subject of obesity. I critique the biomedical approach that reduces the digestive system to a functioning state, similar to that of plumbing. In *Metaphors We Live By*, George Lakoff and Mark Johnson see the house as a container metaphor as "we are physical beings, bounded and set off from the rest of the world by the surface of our skins, and we experience the rest of the world as outside us."[28] Adopting this metaphor, bodies like houses contain a whole host of functioning pipes and wires to give "life" and remove waste. Hidden within the guts of the home, these functions continue without our attention and, like Leder's aforementioned "dys" appearance, it is only through their dysfunction that they appear to us.

The absurd assemblages perform metonymically, as they "stand in" for either something, which appears or functions in a similar way to what they replace. They indicate a form of action and control from possible external interaction with the stop taps to halt or restrict. Although metonymically referencing the viscera, in certain artworks I could manipulate this to both an "inside" and "outside" reading of the body. These internal-like body parts also appear anthropomorphized, looking like bent limbs. Adopting a similar approach to Sarah Lucas, the terse constructions rely on "concise visual analogy."[29] A "lightness of touch" is integral to my making, utilizing the inherent language of the objects, like a "truth to materials," and not exerting too much "pressure" upon them, thoughts also echoing with Lucas:

> You are in a funny relation of mutual respect with the things you use. You are not the dominator of these materials. It's not a case of ramming your ideas into them, because sooner or later you're going to have to accept that these materials are doing something and if you don't go with that you'll end up with a tight-arsed, mediocre artwork.[30]

It enables the artworks to retain its autonomy, using already existing knowledge of the objects in the world and giving it enough signifying content that draws on a reading of the body, but does not attempt to overtly lead to any specific reading. Primarily, the body is used to read the artworks, in how it interacts with the familiar objects, and the body's status as an axis for perception. We are our bodies, of and in the world, and, as proposed by French philosopher Maurice Merleau-Ponty, we perceive the world with our bodies.[31] Through this manipulation and emphasizing of materials and objects, which exists in the physical realm with us, I use materiality to create a dialogue with our bodies.

A piece that aims to be a body rather than of the body, and unites both the inside and outside, is *Deep Seated Anxiety* (see Figure 6.3) Focusing on the female-centric area of the body, the abdomen, the locale of what makes woman "other," emphasizes the core of the body. Many soft/textile sculptures adopt the traditional craft of toy making, by stuffing an enveloping fabric form, like in the artworks by Annette Messager. Sourcing waste materials, fabric, etc., I, however, adopted a buildup technique to create a form and cover this with wadding and finally lightweight calico. The work references notions of reconstructive surgeries with the surface of the calico covered in "sutures" that attempt to reconcile an excess exterior with a smaller interior. Then on either side, a "running" hand-stitch creates a double circular shape similar to those drawn by the plastic surgeon when "targeting" the areas in need of liposuction. This sculpture, and the others like it, does not just rely on the form to connote body, but it is the power of their softness that evokes a bodily empathy. Briony Fer states that soft sculpture invites "a language of anthropomorphism, of bodily projection and empathy. Bulbous forms, organic forms, seemed deliberately to inscribe erotics of the body."[32] I think it is also what it is made from, as mentioned before—the power of textiles resides within its intimate relationship with the body stemming from touch and proximity.

The sensual capacity of textiles contributes to how some of my artworks produce and transmit affect. The bodily projection and empathy, as described by Fer above, works precognitively, reluctantly using a mind/body split—the body has the experience first; the mind follows to cognize such an experience and then tries to put this into vocabulary. Teresa Brennan argues that Western schemas seek to degrade bodily intelligence, putting intellect first, and "that the sense and flesh embody a logic that moves far faster than thought."[33] The fishing hook's penetration in *Forlorn* (see Figure 6.4) creates a bodily empathy, drawing on a similitude between our own sheathing membranes of skin with that of the calico that represents the skin. The site of this piercing also furthers the experience, as it creates an affective transmission, a visceral response in which bodily attention is intensified at the core, or crudely put, "a gut reaction." Affective potential is explained by our own physical being in the physical world, as described by art critic Simon O'Sullivan:

> It is that which connects us to the world. It is the matter in us responding and resonating with the matter around us. . . . This is art's function: to switch our intensive register, to reconnect us with the world. Art opens us up to the non-human universe that we are part of.[34]

The mimetic nature of the anthropomorphic artworks also relates to the body drawing on an empathy of "that being like me" idea and is what Brennan would describe as a transmission of affect brought on through the sense of sight.[35] The mimesis of stretch marks, intestines, and suggestive anthropomorphic stomach-like forms allows viewers to register and locate the relative sites upon their own bodies.

The ambiguity of my artworks oscillates in their readings; while mainly visceral, they may also cause a humorous, repellent, or intriguing reaction. Artist Doris Salcedo states that the power of affect is it "makes art compelling without dictating in what way viewers will be affected."[36] In discussions I had with some viewers of my artworks, I noted their reluctant disclosure of confessing to involuntarily laughing at some artworks. In particular, it was toward the Deviant Bodies series (See Figure 6.5), the orifice-like performative sculptures scattered around

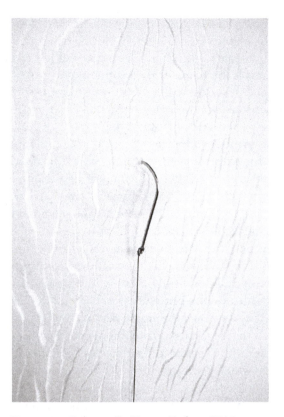

Figure 6.4 Rebecca D. Harris, *Forlorn*, 2013.
(Courtesy of Rebecca D. Harris)

a room, on the floor, animating themselves by giving some sense of being sneaky and mischievous as they seem to explore their location. I became interested in the viewer's reluctance to divulge their experience.

Notably within the current art scene, David Shrigley is best known as the artist who makes "funny" art. At the time of writing this, Shrigley was nominated for the Turner Prize (2013) for his exhibition, which I saw at the Hayward Gallery at the end of 2012. Defending her selection, Penelope Curtis, director of Tate Britain, states that Shrigley's work has been marginalized and overlooked for what has been described as "just funny."[37] Some artworks are funny, but as I will now explain below, humor does not disparage them. In *Art and Laughter* Sheri Klein argues that, since the 1980s, art "has a cynicism that does not lend itself to humor [mainly addressing] political and social issues, but rare is the work that both critiques and makes us smile or laugh."[38] She continues: the aesthetic pleasure normally derived from contemporary artworks stems from its tactility and how an artist uses materials and ideas that can induce "states of awe, puzzlement, melancholy or even

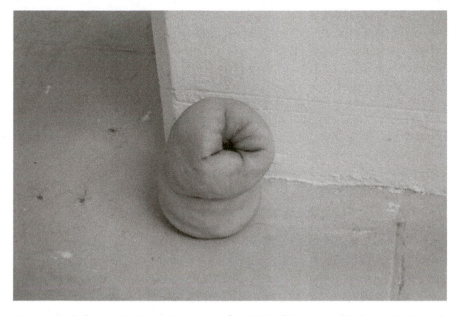

Figure 6.5 Rebecca D. Harris, *Deviant Bodies*, 2013. (Courtesy of Rebecca D. Harris)

repulsion."[39] I position my artworks as attempting any one of the above detailed by Klein, as my artworks oscillate in their readings and, as previously noted by Salcedo, affect does not determine in what ways viewers will be affected.

When considering the subtle humor present in my previous artworks I was initially concerned about making yet another "obese spectacle," like in John Isaacs's satiric sculptures; I naively saw humor as just "making fun" of something. Isaacs's artworks default all too easily to the mockery of the fat body and so is the tendency within popular culture. My apprehension was soon quashed, seeing satire as just one aspect of humor, and to create humorous works, within the theme of fat, it could be intelligently approached and the fat body not automatically caricatured. Klein[40] describes the major theoretical strands of humor as incongruity, psychodynamic, superiority, relief, and sociological, and the forms as parody, pun, paradox, satire, and irony. The major aspects of my own artworks mainly draw on the theory of incongruity through the form of visual puns. Incongruity theory gives a jolt of surprise and then pleasure, stemming from an encounter with something unexpected.[41] The juxtaposition of materials and transposed objects give my artworks the potential to arouse humor. An explanation for this can be sourced as far back as the 1600s from French philosopher Blaise Pascal, who notes, "Nothing produces humor more than a disproportion between that which one expects and that which one sees."[42] Unlike the social theoretical strand of humor,[43] which relies on a shared cultural experience "to get" the joke, incongruity theory, as demonstrated in Pascal's 400-year-old explanation, pervades time and culture. Furthermore, jokes have anonymity, notes Sigmund Freud,[44] and can exist with no knowledge of its producer. This explains the capacity my artworks have for their autonomy, that their "story" is not an essential ingredient for experiencing or reading them. Artworks that induce laughter create a dynamic process between artwork and viewer, who then become intrigued into finding out more about the artwork and why it made them laugh.[45] This is where the "story" can then intersect, and as I stated right already, I aim for my artworks to have a covert approach within the subject matter of obesity.

Throughout this project I seemed to experience varying degrees of fears: fear of "coming out" as fat, fear of having my artworks rejected through associated stigmatized subject matter, and then the fear that "letting" them be funny somehow would undermine them. Although I have overcome much of this fear, it still remains ever so slightly. It is especially the case in fat shaming that my body has been scrutinized my whole life, and although it continues to do so, at least my attention and attitude toward such external impacts have changed. I started my MA degree ignoring my body, and finished by placing it as the axis around which my whole arts practice revolves. Rather, the obese body was a sort of literal elephant in the room, and now forms the crux of my inquiry. I am still anxious about how the artworks and my "coming out" as a fat woman will be received, knowing all too well the negative and sometimes aggressive responses toward fat subjects. Nevertheless, I have grown stronger as an individual, empowered by counterdiscourse and aware that my physical existence need not be "attacked" by others. Contributing to, and encouraging audience engagement with, current debates and other disciplines' research on obesity, I am working on developing collaborative projects with fat activists and leading medical obesity experts. During the time of my project, and financially supported through Plymouth University's equality and diversity grant, I also started contributing research papers to interdisciplinary conferences and I aim for this to continue. The feedback for this has been very encouraging and has highlighted a niche in fat activism for my artworks and written outputs. Although my body became the personal instigator to the project, it later evolved to be of wider significance, no pun intended. Developing the methodological approach of autoethnography, I could use my autobiographical for much wider cultural significance.

NOTES

1. Carolyn Ellis, Tony E. Adams, and Arthur P. Bochner, "Autoethnography: An Overview" *Forum: Qualitative Social Research* 12, no. 1 (2011), accessed May 20, 2013, http://www.qualitative-research.net/index.php/fqs/article/view/1589/3095.

2. Ibid.

3. Drew Leder, *The Absent Body* (Chicago: University of Chicago Press, 1990).

4. Paisley Livingston, *Art and Intention: A Philosophical Study* (Oxford: Oxford University Press, 2005), 209.

5. Eve Sedgwick quoted in Samantha Murray, "(Un/Be) Coming Out? Rethinking Fat Politics," *Social Semiotics* 15, no. 2 (2006): 157.

6. Murray, "(Un/Be) Coming Out?," 155.

7. Samantha Murray, *The Fat Female Body* (Basingstoke: Palgrave Macmillan, 2008), 4–5.

8. Gillian Rose, *Visual Methodologies: An Introduction to Researching with Visual Material* (London: Sage, 2012), 190.

9. Sara Mills, *Michel Foucault* (London: Routledge, 2003), 55–56.

10. Julia Twigg, "Clothing, Age and the Body: A Critical Review," *Ageing & Society*, 27 (2007): 28, accessed May 19, 2013, http://www.kent.ac.uk/sspssr/staff/academic/twigg/clothing-age-body.pdf.

11. Ibid.

12. Claudia Benthien, *Skin: On the Cultural Border between Self and the World* (New York: Columbia University Press, 2002).

13. Rozsika Parker, *The Subversive Stitch: Embroidery and the Making of the Feminine* (New York: I. B. Tauris, 2010).

14. Senga Negundi, in Anne Wagner, "Sarah Lucas: Ordinary Language and Bodily Magic," *Sarah Lucas: Ordinary Things*, exhibition held at the Henry Moore Institute, United Kingdom, July–October 2012 [exhibition catalogue] (2012): 51.

15. Murray, "(Un/Be) Coming Out?," 154–55.

16. Leder, *The Absent Body*, 93–95.

17. Murray, *The Fat Female Body*, 91.

18. Ibid.

19. Ibid.

20. Benthien, *Skin*, 86.

21. Ibid.

22. Ibid., 86–87.

23. Ibid., 14.

24. Rachel A. J. Hurst, "Tracing the Skin's Surface: From Psychoanalysis to the Television Makeover," *Octopus: Surface* 4 (2008): 115, accessed January 20, 2013, http://www.theoctopusjournal.org/storage/volume-4/Octo_Vol4_2008_Surface_Hurst_pages103-123.pdf.

25. Claire Pajackowska, "Tension, Time and Tenderness: Indexical Traces of Touch in Textiles," in *Digital and Other Virtualities. New Encounters: Arts, Cultures, Concepts*, ed. Antony Bryant and Griselda Pollock (London: I. B. Tauris, 2010), 10, accessed February 20, 2012, http://researchonline.rca.ac.uk/917/1/Indexical_traces_of_touch.pdf.

26. Bill Hughes, "Medicalized Bodies," in *The Body, Culture and Society: An Introduction* (Buckingham: Open University Press, 2000), 16–17.

27. Ibid.

28. George Lakoff and Mark Johnson, *Metaphors We Live By* (Chicago: University of Chicago Press, 2003), 29.

29. Jan Van Adrichem, *Sarah Lucas* [exhibition catalogue], exhibition held at Museum Boymans Van Beuningen, Rotterdam, February–March 1996, (1996): 9.

30. Ibid., 10.

31. Maurice Merleau-Ponty, *Phenomenology of Perception* (London: Routledge, 2005).

32. Briony Fer, "Objects beyond Objecthood," *Oxford Art Journal* 22, no. 2 (1999): 29, accessed April 15, 2013, http://www.jstor.org/stable/1360633.

33. Teresa Brennan, *The Transmission of Affect* (Ithaca, NY: Cornell University Press, 2004), 136.

34. Simon O'Sullivan, "The Aesthetics of Affect: Thinking Art beyond Representation," *Angelaki: Journal of the Theoretical Humanities* 6, no. 3 (2001): 125–35.

35. Brennan, *The Transmission of Affect*, 56.

36. Doris Salcedo, in Mieke Bal, *Of What One Cannot Speak: Doris Salcedo's Political Art* (Chicago: University of Chicago Press, 2010), 3.

37. Penelope Curtis in Charlotte Higgins, "Turner Prize 2013: A Shortlist Strong on Wit and Charm," *Guardian*, April 25, 2013, accessed May 20, 2013, http://www.guardian.co.uk/artanddesign/2013/apr/25/turner-prize-2013-shortlist1.

38. Sheri Klein, *Art and Laughter* (London: I. B. Tauris, 2007), 27.

39. Ibid.

40. Ibid.

41. Ibid.

42. Blaise Pascal in Klein, *Art and Laughter*, 10.

43. Klein, *Art and Laughter*.

44. Sigmund Freud, *Jokes and Their Relation to the Unconscious* (London: Vintage Books, 2001), 142.

45. Klein, *Art and Laughter*, 27.

7

A Bigger Tent

Nancy Ellis-Ordway

Ashley, at 17, has finally agreed with her mother that she needs treatment for her anxiety. She is slender and conventionally pretty. After a couple of counseling sessions to get to know each other, I begin talking with her about anxiety management techniques. We talk about what it means to "take a deep breath." I instruct her how to breathe deeply into her belly. Her eyes widen. "You mean, let my stomach get all distended?" she asks. Yes, I say, that's exactly what I mean. "Will it be permanent?" she gasps.

Most of the discourse in the Fat Acceptance Movement has been, understandably, focused on the lived experience of fat people. The impact of that observed experience on nonfat people has often been overlooked or ignored. Addressing this oversight has powerful implications for people of all sizes.

My background is in therapy rather than research or activism, and I have been treating people with eating disorders and body image issues for 30 years. I have watched how the "war on obesity" has changed the way people think and feel about their bodies. While it is certainly true that people of size are much more likely to be bullied and vilified about their weight, thinner people do not escape unscathed. However, thinner people are not only left out of the conversation; many of them don't even know there *is* a conversation. If we want a massive, culture-wide shift in attitudes about weight and health, we must acknowledge that the current attitudes negatively affect *everybody*, not just folks who are above a certain body mass index.

When I started working in this field, the "typical" eating disordered patient was a teenage girl who had been chubby, started a diet, received positive attention for her weight loss, and then got carried away. Over the last decade or so, I have increasingly seen individuals who have always been slender, but who are so terrified by the idea of becoming fat that they have developed symptoms that meet the diagnostic criteria for anorexia or bulimia nervosa. Frequently, the trigger was a lecture in a health class about the dangers of becoming fat, or a comment from a health care professional about weight control. The terror of all the negative consequences of weight gain drives restrictive and disordered eating.

In the arsenal of the war on obesity, the most potent weapon is shame. There is a widespread misapprehension that enough shame will motivate fat people to lose weight. Shame does not lead to positive behavior change; it only leads to body loathing and self-hate. Shame is like a poisonous gas: it affects the intended victim but it also spreads and infects anyone in the general vicinity. Whether shaming is inadvertent or deliberate, the effect is devastating. Shaming anyone for his or her body size is wrong and should be stopped, not only because of the negative effect it has on the intended target but also because of the damage it does to everyone else. Television shows such as *The Biggest Loser* serve as cautionary tales to slender individuals as well: "Be very careful or you too could end up like this! And that would be the worst thing that could possibly happen!"

Recently, I was in a classroom setting and heard the comment "Yes, we know that efforts to lose weight don't work, so what is important is to not get fat in the first place." The speaker believed that she was voicing a gentler idea that she thought would reduce the stigma on people already fat, but the implications are not that simple. First, it dismisses fat people as hopeless, and second, it raises the expectations on the nonfat to be extra vigilant about their weight, to be sure it doesn't creep upward. I have read variations of this comment in other places during recent years, and while I appreciate the effort to decrease the blame placed on fat people, I think it is destructive on a whole new level.

Hunger, appetite, eating, and satisfaction are at the core of our earliest experiences in infancy. How we satisfy our hunger is an intensely intimate and personal activity that we engage in several times a day. When we believe that we cannot be trusted to make good decisions about what we eat, when we are told that we must follow an external set of rules to make sure we don't eat too much, we lose trust in our competence to make choices in other areas of our lives as well. We lose faith in the inherent wisdom of our bodies.

Body dissatisfaction is the new normal. When people of all sizes come to me for therapy, regardless of the presenting problem, many of them eventually talk about a deep sense of body shame. This shame combines with a distrust of the body, which is never what it is "supposed" to be. Appetite for food cannot be trusted and therefore the self cannot be trusted.

Quality of life suffers when the preoccupation with limiting food intake becomes the focus. The emphasis on food restriction crowds out possibilities for social interaction, relationships, and accomplishments. When food is regarded as dangerous, the ability to enjoy eating erodes. At the same time, comments like "I shouldn't be eating this," or "I'll have to run an extra mile tomorrow to work this off," or even "I stayed at the gym an extra hour today so I could have this meal with you," are so common as to be unremarkable. Comments like these reflect a distrust of the body and a sense of shame about its appetites. These comments interfere with the natural enjoyment of eating, both for the person talking and for anyone listening. At the same time, this attitude in naturally slender people is not contributing to their slenderness, only to their body dissatisfaction.

Preoccupation with achieving or maintaining a lower weight has negative effects on emotional and physical health. Restrictive eating can result in deficiencies of nutrients essential to healthy functioning. Weight focus can lead some individuals to avoid the physical activity necessary for cardiovascular fitness if it results in increased appetite but not weight loss. Limiting intake to less than what the body needs leads to preoccupation with food. I have learned to ask, "What percentage of your day do you spend thinking about food and eating?" The answer is often "Oh, all the time!"—regardless of the size of the person speaking. I then ask, "How might your life be different if you only spent 20 or 30 percent of your time thinking about food?" Often, that is unimaginable. The extra time and energy could be used relaxing, connecting with loved ones, making new friends, starting a new hobby, or even thinking about ways to change the world.

The war on obesity is predicated on the idea that causing shame and guilt for eating will result in weight loss and improved health for those who are deemed "too heavy." Not only does this not lead to sustained weight loss; it leads to unhealthy weight cycling and to ever-increasing levels of internalized body loathing in people of all sizes. Shaming messages toward fat people in the media and culture impact those of lower weights by making them terrified of having those messages aimed at them. Human beings are designed to enjoy the activity of eating. We take pleasure in preparing, serving, sharing, and consuming food when we are adequately nourished on a regular basis. Undereating and shame about eating destroy that pleasure, depriving people of all sizes of something that should be a source of joy.

Not long ago I was involved in a discussion about eating in which a well-educated gentleman made a comment about "those times when someone *should* feel guilty about eating." Due to time constraints, I was unable to respond to him, but it made me wonder about times when guilt about eating might be appropriate. If I work in an office and I steal someone else's lunch out of the refrigerator, I should feel guilty about eating it. If I eat the last piece of cantaloupe that I know my son was saving for breakfast, I should feel guilty. If I am an Orthodox Jew and I eat pork, it may be appropriate to feel guilty. The only examples I could come up with in which guilt would be a reasonable response to eating involves stolen food or violation of religious beliefs. The prevailing belief in the current fat-phobic culture, however, is that guilt about any and all eating is necessary and desirable.

How we experience being in our bodies is also impacted by a negative focus on body size. As a body-oriented therapist, I consider breath to be of central importance. How we breathe impacts how we feel and how we function in life. I often talk about the neurobiology of anger and fear in my work with individuals and couples as well as in a continuing education class in safety awareness training. For several years I have been asking people to take a deep breath and let me watch them. I have come to the conclusion that the only people in our culture who breathe correctly are singers, wind instrument players, and yoga practitioners. The cultural imperative of "Suck in your gut! Don't let your belly hang out!" has created constricted breathing, resulting in higher levels of anxiety and a chronic inability to relax in the population at large. Again, this affects people of all sizes.

Several years ago, a young couple came to me for marriage counseling. They were in their late twenties, both slender and attractive in the conventional sense. The woman I estimated to be a size 6, a size 8 at the most. They identified their problem as an inability to discuss much of anything without getting into a screaming match. After getting some background information, I began explaining about what happens in the brain when the fight/flight/freeze response is triggered and how it becomes difficult to think or talk rationally. When I got to the part about taking a deep breath, the woman became quite agitated. "I can't do that!" she exclaimed. "I can't let my stomach get big like that!" At this point the husband nearly came out of his seat. "Do you see that?" he yelled at me. "Do you see what I put up with?" He went on to say that she wouldn't let him see her naked, or let him touch her belly or thighs. He interpreted this as rejection, but she was so lost in her own body shame that she could not consider how it affected her relationship. Unfortunately, they canceled their second appointment and I don't know what the outcome was for them.

I hear variations on this theme frequently from people who come to me for therapy. Certainly, there are some people in the world who make obnoxious comments to their partners about weight, but I think there are many more who are just bewildered by the body shame and self-hatred in their partners. Intimacy, both physical and emotional, erodes over time, and the relationship suffers. Responses to expression of body dissatisfaction usually focus on weight loss. "Well then, if you feel bad about your weight, let's go on a diet together. Let's go to the gym." This attempt at support usually backfires, because no amount of change in the body will result in increased body love; instead it reinforces the idea of the body and its appetites as the enemy. Unfortunately, guidelines for learning how to love one's body exactly the way it is today are drowned out by the messages that the body is unacceptable and needs to change.

Fat acceptance is a social justice movement. The concept of "a big enough tent" refers to expanding the boundaries of a group to include more people, more viewpoints, and more ideas. When fat acceptance is talked about only by fat people, the larger culture finds it easy to dismiss. True widespread fat acceptance would benefit everyone by encouraging an appreciation of body and size diversity, allowing people of all sizes to love and trust their own bodies regardless of size.

Other social justice movements that focus on human rights involve "allies," individuals who believe in a cause that does not directly affect them. As a Caucasian, straight, cisgender woman, I can be an "ally" in the struggle against racism or homophobia, but neither of those affect me directly. I can be aware of my own privilege while I stand up for people who are mistreated simply because I think it is the right thing to do. "Thin allies" in the fat acceptance movement are aware of thin privilege, but most of them are also aware of how they have been personally affected by weight stigma and body hatred. I believe that there are no "allies" in fat acceptance, because we are all in this together.

As long as the fat acceptance movement focuses only on the way that weight stigma affects fat people, we are excluding a large segment of the population who could be involved. However, individuals who have been bullied and mistreated all their lives for being fat are unlikely to be very sympathetic to the woes of terrified skinny people. Certainly, weight stigma carries its most severe consequences for those who are large, but that does not diminish the negative impact on everyone else. It makes me think of the adage "I wept because I had no shoes until I met a man who had no feet." Even when I was a child, this idea irritated me but it took me years to be able to articulate why: Yes, it is very sad that there are individuals who have no feet. That does not mean that we should ignore the plight of the shoeless. Being shoeless is also unfortunate and may have serious consequences. How bad does shoelessness have to be before it deserves consideration? Is one adult homeless person in a city important enough to have someone make an effort to provide shoes? What about a first grader in Boise or Minneapolis in January?

Finding shoes for the shoeless will not help the person with no feet, but acknowledging the impact of weight stigma on the nonfat will ultimately benefit fat people by engaging more voices in the efforts to create a weight-neutral culture. If large people are the casualties in the war on obesity, thin people are the hostages.

8

Dating While Fat: One Fierce Fat Girl's Experience

Jeanette Miller

The phrase "dating sucks" is an age-old adage for a reason. Put two people with expectations for a good time together, regardless of their short- or long-term intentions, and it sounds like tons of fun. Now let's factor in body insecurity, personal baggage, emotional scars, and the hard life that can come with the soft cushions of a fat body, and there's bound to be some pitfalls. I'm not saying that people don't enjoy dates; they do. Fat people do. I do. But it's a formula fraught with the potential for disaster and yet it's Western societies' structural standard for how two people "should" meet and get to know each other before commencing whatever type of consensual relationship they are in search of.

As I think about being fat and dating, I'm struck by what readers might wonder about how my personal dating history has anything to do with the politics of size and fat acceptance. Well, a person's story is important and often critical to developing a full understanding of their motivations for how they move through life. I'm fat. I've always been fat. I consider myself a fat activist. I'm also a feminist. A fabulously fierce fat feminist. "Dating" is a term I use as an "umbrella" that covers all things from meeting for coffee, casual sex, and nonexclusive shared time with a person or people of one's choosing, to sharing time together with fully committed exclusivity to a single individual. While I consider myself to be heteroflexible, I make the choice here to write primarily about heterosexual dating. It's where the bulk of my experience is and where my journey to self and size acceptance has been most influenced. My feminism informs my fat activism and requires that I live the same life principles that I dedicate most of my professional work and personal passions to. That includes owning all the rights, responsibilities, obligations, and consequences of my body and how I use it. As a fat activist, I believe that every

BODY should be treated equally. I haven't always accepted my fat body and I certainly haven't always been open to exposing my fat body, metaphorically or physically, to someone else while dating. And yet, dating in its various forms has influenced the journey to full acceptance of my body as it is at this moment in time.

My dating story starts at an early age. My adolescent body was a size that now, as a reasonable adult, I would consider to be "average." Yet I was still larger than everyone else in my fifth-grade class when I met the boy who would be my first boyfriend—we rode a four-wheeler, my arms wrapped tightly around his waist, through the bean fields we were supposed to be weeding during summer vacation and had our first kiss on the Ferris wheel at the county fair. My first sexual experience occurred at the age of 13 with the smallest boy in class, in my parents' basement bedroom. The years that followed were a mix of adolescent/teen heartbreak, summer flings with the sheriff's nephew, pregnancy scares, skinny dipping with the guys at the lake, and smoking pot while getting drunk under the stars in the cemetery. I was always the biggest girl in the group, and while the other "skinnier" girls were putting out to almost every guy in class (we went to a small school), I preferred a steady guy who gave me his full attention. It felt safer knowing that this person had seen my body and hadn't rejected me because of it. I put on a significant amount of weight during my high school years and, growing increasingly uncomfortable with myself and my sexuality, I stopped dating. My favorite guy-friend in high school made out with me in his car during lunch and referred to me as his "little sister" while hanging out at the lockers with the boys. This was the first time I remember experiencing someone else being embarrassed by the size of my body to the point where he wouldn't acknowledge the true nature of our relationship. It felt shameful.

For a lot of years during my early adulthood, I also didn't date. I'd hang out with friends and do social things in groups, from time to time hooking up with someone else once a certain level of comfort set in. This felt like a really safe way to spend time with men, and while my body disgusted me, I was still interested in socializing. Although self-hatred caused me to shut down emotionally, I did not shut out or hide from the world. As a dear friend recently told me, "You are this strange mix of social butterfly and emotional introvert." I know that this personality trait became most fully developed around this time as a protective mechanism against how I felt about myself, was treated in the real world, and the contradictions that sex and physical attraction brought into my life.

In my late twenties while I was graduating from university and coming out of a long-distance relationship, I met this amazing man, a soldier. We were fast friends and remained just that for well over a year. As a friend, he was very encouraging about my appearance. Always chastised me for putting myself down and always told me I was beautiful. When we started dating and our feelings grew, he was very adamant about loving me for me. He shot down any idea for diets or new exercise regimens and instead assured me that he thought I was sexy. He never used the word "fat" or phrases like "large body," only "your body." He encouraged me to embrace it and love it as much as he did. I knew he loved me, but I always doubted that he loved my body too. We had a couple of great years together when he went to fight the war in Afghanistan and didn't make it back alive. It was eight years before I seriously considered trusting both my heart and body to a man again in the way I had with him. I dated and hooked up, both in search of ways to heal from the pain of loss and with the desire to feel good about myself like I did sometimes when I was with him. I didn't understand that feeling could only truly come from inside myself and that it would mean spending time *with* myself, about seven years to be exact before I knew how the best love of all—self-acceptance—felt.

Acceptance of my body, as is, did not happen overnight and it didn't begin with dating. After graduate school, I started a new job at a prestigious university, and within just a few years, I was recognized for both my skills and talents and received multiple promotions. My self-confidence grew and I became emboldened. The second job I took exposed me fully to my true passions of feminism and activism and I dived in head first to the size acceptance movement with a deep breath, trusting that I would surface a better person. I learned a lot from others about loving my body as it is and dressing in fashionable clothing in ways that made me feel attractive and confident. I saw happy fat people in love with other fat and not so fat people. And I began to carry myself with more confidence and self-assurance than ever before. I wasn't a better person; I was the me I was intended to be all along. And all of that came to fruition without a single date, but not without the support and encouragement of amazing friends and a strong community.

Then one day a friend I'd known for several years told me that his long-term relationship was open and asked if I might be interested in getting to know him more intimately. And so I entered into a very safe and comfortable situation. Were we dating? By the broad definition of this chapter, yes. We were in a relationship, nonexclusive and yet very loving. He was not my "type" at all, but I adored his quiet nerdiness and disturbing sense of humor. Plus he knew me. He'd seen me in my pajamas with unkempt hair and dirty teeth many times from sleeping over at their house and yet he was still interested in me. This happened right around the same time that I discovered self-acceptance and unapologetic love for my body. Not a coincidence. I asked him once why after so many years of friendship he decided to make the move to something more intimate. His answer was that he'd sensed something change in me. He couldn't place it, but it showed in the way I carried myself and was now moving through life. It was confidence and no longer feeling the need to apologize for my mere existence.

At this point in my life and my self-acceptance journey, this was the ideal dating relationship for me. I'm sure some of you will either shake your head in disapproval, be vaguely disturbed by the prospect, or possibly be slightly envious. Open relationships aren't for everyone and they can be a significant challenge. But what I appreciated about it were the very clear rules and expectations. He and his partner had rules for what happened in and out of the relationship. No sex in their house. No falling in love. While I was the secondary person he saw most often, he also saw other people from time to time. I needed to be okay with that, without doubting that he still cared about me very much. It was nice to know what to expect. He clearly liked me, was attracted to my mind and body, and I didn't need to second-guess where this relationship would go. It was comfortable and freeing. This newfound freedom in a dating relationship gave me the leeway to explore my own boundaries between size acceptance, dating, relationships, physicality, and sex. For the first time, I walked around completely, comfortably naked in front of someone I was dating. I didn't try to cover up or wear clothes. I would get up and get something out of the kitchen without grabbing a robe and I didn't get shy when I caught him watching me; and he loved to watch me. I loved that. The fact that my fat body, which I also now was accepting of, was desirable to him that he wanted me just as I am, was intoxicating. And it wasn't just about sex. We went out to eat and to movies. While we shopped during the holidays for gifts for his partner, I got ideas on what he'd want in his stocking. When we were out together, he'd hold my hand and kiss me. His treatment of me both publicly and privately were very much the same. He wasn't ashamed to be seen, intimately, with me in public. It was the first time in my life I experienced this without doubt. The relationship ended about nine months later. The circumstances were unavoidable and mostly amicable. Although we are still very close friends, he and his partner now live in a different state. We text regularly and talk occasionally. I'm grateful for our time together and sometimes desperately miss the comfort and acceptance I felt around him. But if you asked me today if I would be happy in that type of relationship, I would likely say no. Because the more I grew to love myself within the safeness of that relationship, the more I knew I not only wanted more, but I also deserved more. After healing my bruised heart, I welcomed the opportunity to move forward with full gusto back into the dating scene.

As I think most single women my age would attest, today's dating scene is in stark contrast to a comfortable relationship. It's unpredictable, gritty, and you really do have to kiss a lot of frogs. What men are looking for when they ask a woman out falls within a wide range and of course they aren't typically direct or even honest about it. My experience with dating revealed that there were a lot of men looking mostly for sex without a commitment of time or self. I think this is true within most communities with various sizes of people. I wouldn't say it's unique to being fat. Although it also was clear that while these men were clearly attracted to me, they were also still experiencing the pressure of society, friends, family to date within the "norm" instead of dating a fat woman they are actually more attracted to. Early on, I was meeting most of these men in a club I danced at regularly on the weekends. My confidence and newfound sexual identity definitely made me more attractive to men, and I frequently took home numbers from two or three men on any given Saturday night. About one out of every three of the individuals attached to those numbers actually followed through by answering their phone when I called or by calling me. Only about half of those then wanted to meet me again in person. A good majority of them were interested only in sex. To be fair, I was willing. I was feeling myself—I liked what I saw looking back at me in the mirror. I was big, beautiful, and hella sexy; of course I was going to enjoy that ride. But they rarely called back and second dates were even more scarce. As I began to notice that some of these men were unwilling to be seen in public with me outside of the local BBW club, I was reminded of the shame I felt at a younger age when similar things happened. But I was stronger now. I held to one standard—they had to meet me in public first. As a feminist activist of size, I wasn't going be hidden away by men I knew desired me in private but were publicly ashamed of me. I thought insisting that we be out in public together would change this. The dates were fun; we always had a good time. But then, suddenly, they would take a steep nosedive when they would stop calling or wouldn't respond to a text. These men who one minute were really enjoying my company were like ghosts the following day, as if they never actually existed. I was shocked by how that could be. Was disappearing really easier or better than telling someone you weren't interested anymore or than dealing with whatever ridicule you might experiencing by actually sticking by someone you are attracting to? It seemed so.

I grew really tired of the games of the dating world, frequently sharing my frustration with friends who would suggest different places to meet men who might behave differently. I was encouraged to hold men to a higher standard, to not have sex with them, if they were treating me this way. As much as I wanted a solid relationship, I also really liked sex and I wasn't giving up sex to wait around for a man who can't handle the pressure that often comes with dating a fat girl. I know there are supposed "rules" about how soon in relationship to have sex, who should call after the first date and within how many days, and such nonsense, but those seemed so arbitrary and nonsensical. Why couldn't I just have sex when and with whomever I wanted to? Did I need a relationship? Didn't I own this body I was so accepting of now? Didn't I make the decisions for its pleasure? So, I made a conscious decision to throw out all the rule books (even though I didn't own any) about how women are supposed to behave in respect to men and relationships. There would be no rules for me and I would model my interactions with men off the way some men had treated me—there was no need to spend time with them in public if we were both only after sex. If, like in the movies, a man could pick up a woman at the grocery store, take her home for hot sex, and send her on her way before her perishables went bad, then why couldn't I do this in real life? The answer, of course, was that I could. I absolutely could. And I did. Well, I didn't go to the grocery store. Not the grocery store, because I hate grocery shopping . . . but most of their home delivery drivers are men, *wink.* I picked up the barista who'd been flirting with me for months after work one night and he made me coffee the next morning, in my apartment. I'd meet men out and about and would take them home with me. A guy I had been attracted to in the club, but knew to be a player, soon became a lover once I accepted that I didn't need to see him anywhere else than in my bedroom. Confidence in my body fed my ego and I began to enjoy being the proverbial player. But while my sexual confidence and physical pleasure improved with each encounter, my emotional confidence and desire to feel the love and acceptance I'd once experienced in a relationship were suffering. I blew off friends' suggestions that my revolving door was a protective device. That I was afraid to let someone love me, or worse yet, to let myself have feelings for someone else. And they were right. I had thought that loving myself and body would mean I would finally be perfectly happy, and knowing that there were men who actually wanted to be with ME, fat body and all, had made me believe that I actually would find that proverbial happy ever after. And when I didn't, I filled the void with empty pleasure and men who were certainly not deserving of my time or energy. I felt like all the work I'd done to love myself as a complete person, mind and body, was for naught. Maybe I did need some rules after all.

So now, I'm switching up my approach to dating. I've started giving men a chance (sometimes more than one and occasionally more than they deserve) to show me that they are in it for more than access to my body. And I've stopped using them for their body. I've decided I'm ready for more and absolutely not willing to settle for less. Because whether society (and sometimes myself) believes it or not, as a fat girl, I'm allowed to have standards and expectations. It feels like it's been a long journey. I learned some things I thought I already knew, and looking back I can see both where being a feminist and size acceptance activist informed my decisions in ways that were helpful and where I used these two parts of my core to support behavior that harmed me and sometimes others. Self-acceptance, especially around size, is not an easy journey. And when we throw in the myriad of different types of relationships—friends, family, lovers, strangers, coworkers, society at large—that we are irrevocably connected to, it sometimes gets messy. And I'm not even close to having a solution for that. But here's what I know for sure: "The Rules" of dating and relationships, whichever ones you've read in shiny magazines or self-help books, weren't written for and don't apply to really anyone, but especially not to someone on a journey of size acceptance. Society is fucked up and society's "rules" around policing bodies are absolutely meant to be broken. The only rules you should even consider following are the ones you make for yourself; and only you can decide if they should be broken. My journey, in particular this path of dating while fat (and become fat accepting), has informed the creation of my own rules. Your journey will inform yours. I share mine here only as an example of what I have found to be most crucial to preserving myself, my self-love, and my love of others along the way.

THIS ONE FAT GIRL'S RULES FOR HAPPY DATING AND A FABULOUS LIFE

Rule 1: Love and accept yourself (mind, soul, and body) as you are in this moment, first. And most. Let me be clear. I'm not selfish. I don't recommend selfishness. But I do have to love myself before I can love someone else. This includes accepting and loving the body I live in here and now. Again, well-known adages. Because they ring true. Loving and accepting myself allows me to be confident and comfortable with others. Also, love myself most, because if I love someone more than I love myself, I am at risk of losing myself in the relationship.

Rule 2: Don't settle for someone who won't take you out (to dinner, to the movies, to walk through a park or a flea market). It's not about spending money; it's about being seen in public. It's about them saying in a very public way, without words, "I like/love this fat girl and want everyone to know it." And bonus-activist-moment, because you are breaking out of the expectations society has for you and him. It's a big FU to anyone who thinks fat girls shouldn't be seen, let alone appreciated for exactly who they are. And it will be reassuring to the fat girl who's there by herself, on her own journey.

Rule 3: When something feels important, ask for it. Compromise? Yes. But I can't get what I want if I don't ask. And I likely won't know what they want either. I know as fats, this goes against everything we've ever learned about staying out of the way, not asking for anything we need/want, apologizing for our existence. But I'm going to ask, negotiate, and compromise. And then I'm going to follow through and hold the other person accountable too.

Rule 4: Stay strong. Don't fold. I deserve to be loved and accepted for who I am. I deserve to be someone else's priority when I make them mine.

I deserve respect. I won't settle for less and I won't give in when that is all I'm offered.

Rule 5: I won't let my fear of being alone make me settle for something less than what I want, need, and deserve. There is someone meant to love me the way I need them to.

Rule 6: Have fun and don't take myself too seriously. Every day is a new day. I want to have as few regrets as possible. So I laugh a lot. And I take chances.

After all I've experienced, one thing really does ring true for me. Dating does suck. It sucks your energy, time, and sometimes your self-esteem. And when you are on a journey to unapologetic self-love and size acceptance like I am, you'll be challenged to your very core. How to deal with this, for me, is so dependent on how I feel about myself, and that includes how I feel about my body. So, I choose to continue striving to love and respect all of me, including my body, unapologetically, boldly, and without fear.

9

Bait and Switch: Commodification and Agency in *Diet or Die: The Dolly Dimples Weight Reducing Plan*

Kate Browne

When Celesta Geyer stepped up to the fat lady banner at the Happy Land carnival sideshow, she did not have a clear grasp on what compelled her to do so. The carnival provided a break in the limited, monotonous social activities available for Geyer and her husband, Frank, during Depression-era economic hardship, and she felt drawn to the fat lady banner by "a strange power." After being unexpectedly hailed by the ticket taker to come closer, she challenged him by asking, "Do you want to see a real 338-pound fat lady?" Her question was met with laughter—he explained that Jolly Pearl, the fat lady working inside the tent, was nearly twice as fat. The ticket taker allowed the couple to see the show for free and meet "Jolly" Pearl Stanley, who suggested Geyer join the show as a gimmick. Geyer, the smaller of the two women, would stand outside with the ticket taker who would "tell the crowd that the fat lady inside is twice as fat as the one they see on the platform."[1] Stanley suggested the trick would work because the crowd was skeptical and curious— they would not believe that anyone could be *that* fat. Geyer believed that her body was unusual in the extreme because until this moment, she lived a life mostly isolated from other fat people. Her life experience was shaped by living in a material and cultural world based on the same skepticism that prompted an audience to pay to see the "impossible."

Stanley and Geyer bonded over a shared experience of social isolation and stigma outside the sideshow canvas. Initially, Geyer was not sure if she wanted to take the job over fears that she would upset her husband's ideal of a perfect home and what her family would think of her new line of work. Stanley pressed on. "You know, honey, everyone laughs at you now. Don't you think it would be a good idea to make them pay for their fun?" Geyer considered the opportunity presented by Stanley as an advantageous one but was still discouraged by the thought of putting her body—a body she was ashamed of and previously encouraged to keep hidden—on a public platform. Having never considered the possibility of performing as a fat lady, Geyer finally concluded that she agreed with Stanley: "Of course, I'd like to make them pay. I'd like to make them pay in cash and a thousand different ways."[2]

The fat lady act in the American sideshow—especially one that uses the gimmick described by Geyer—represents the paradoxical relationship between fat bodies, diet culture, and commodification. Behind the curtain, freak show performance presented an opportunity for fat men and women to create a material world free from shame or stigma. Comfortable chairs, clothes, and other goods were made specifically for large bodies. Fat performers who traveled together developed a necessary social community and felt relieved that they could engage in everyday activities like eating in ways they felt were impossible among the general public. Performing in the freak show often provided more income than other working- or middle-class jobs commonly considered appropriate for fat people. On the other hand, the success of the performance relied on stereotypes and the novelty of the fat body as an object of staring and ridicule. Offstage, fat men and women faced the very real, very damaging effects of a material world that refused to accommodate their bodies.

Commodification of female fat bodies is a constant theme in Geyer's 1968 memoir *Diet or Die: The Dolly Dimples Weight Reducing Plan*. From the challenges of finding ready-to-wear clothes to being a consumer of weight loss products to finding work in the sideshow, Celesta "Dolly Dimples" Geyer describes living in a complex world where her fat body is both a shamed object of ridicule and a means to financial independence and social community. Neither Geyer nor her sideshow persona, Dolly Dimples, serves as a heroine for fat women—ultimately, Geyer succumbs to popular ideas of fat as pathology and embarks on the strict weight loss program that provides the somewhat misleading subtitle for the book.[3] Of the memoir's 239 pages, only 40 pages describe the motivation for weight loss and the plan Geyer followed. Like many weight loss memoirs, Geyer also includes a sample weekly menu and recipes intended as a guide for readers searching for weight loss success. The publication of the book marks another point of commodity as the emerging weight loss memoir genre provided her with an additional source of income since she could no longer perform in the sideshow. Although Geyer's book did not do well commercially, book sales for this genre depend on "before-and-after" rhetoric that positions fat bodies as out of control and incomplete.[4]

I choose to read *Diet or Die* as informed by fat studies and feminist disability studies to explore the complicated and problematic relationship of the female fat body to commodification as both a product of and accomplice to the promotion of weight loss as a response to fat stigma. Feminist disability studies views the construction of disability not as personal pathology but as a category similar to race, class, and gender that is informed by social, historical, and cultural influences.[5] In this case, it would be incorrect to conflate disability with physical impairment. Fat bodies become disabled when material realities do not meet the needs of fat people to allow access to public places and spaces. However, fat studies scholars tend to reject the label of fat bodies as disabled because it implies physical impairment or abnormality. I recognize this controversy and the variation of interpretation for fatness in relation to disability, but this piece focuses on material and consumer conditions that disable fat bodies rather than an assumption that the fat body is inherently a disabled one.

Fat studies as an intellectual field of inquiry is a relative newcomer when paired with fields such as feminism, critical race theory, queer theory, and disability studies, but specifically seeks to challenge and analyze medical, legal, and cultural discourses that discriminate against fat people.[6] Incorporating complementary critical approaches does the work of filling gaps in previous scholarship while developing a more robust strategy for emerging methods. Both fat studies and feminist disability studies share the goal of rejecting pathologizing fat bodies and redirect the focus from the deviant individual to historical, cultural, and social effects of structural oppression. I suggest an alternate reading of Diet or Die that acknowledges Geyer's attempts at subverting diet discourse through her employment as a sideshow fat lady in ways other employment could not help her achieve despite ultimately succumbing to the fallacy of weight loss as the preferred solution for coping with fat oppression.

Hillel Schwartz identifies the development of "before-and-after" weight loss discourse beginning in the mid-twentieth century.[7] In this type of narrative, the fat body as "Before" is perceived as disobedient, undesirable, dysfunctional, and barbaric and generally denied existence. The liminal phase of a dieter is always perceived as linear moving toward the "After" body as desirable, controlled, optimal, and civilized. This form is often credited to Weight Watchers founder Jean Nidetch who encouraged members to rely on memory of their existence as a "Before" body as motivation to become and stay an "After." For Nidetch, memory operates in conjunction with visual and material reminders such as carrying a "Before" picture at all times and trying on clothes of the desired "After" size to reinforce the constant vigilance required in dieting.[8] This visual rhetoric is reproduced on the cover of Diet or Die showing Geyer as a "Before" using a promotional show photograph as Dolly Dimples on the left opposite an "After" photograph to the right. The cover for Nidetch's own 1972 weight loss memoir, The Story of Weight Watchers, is almost identical with the title above the photographs depicting "Before" on the left and "After" opposite right.

Rosemarie Garland-Thomson argues that parallels exist in the social construction of female bodies and disabled bodies since "both are defined in opposition to a norm that is assumed to possess natural physical superiority."[9] By extension, fat bodies have also been interpreted as inherently female so gender theory lends itself to similar interpretation of thin/fat descriptors. Just as bodies are marked by male/female binaries, fat bodies are also marked thin/fat, and always on the Before side of before/after. Kathleen LeBesco invokes Judith Butler's theory on performativity, which "requires looking at performances in context and asking, What performance in what context will help destabilize naturalized identity categories."[10] Marked, fat bodies in public constantly perform fat as an identity category, and many anecdotes in weight loss memoirs revolve around negative experiences as a fat body in public. Authors of weight loss memoirs regularly and proudly describe how those same experiences are no longer an issue as a thin body in public. Autobiography becomes a performative act that reasserts thin privilege and discursively unmarks the author's body as fat. Weight loss on its own unmarks only the physical body; so, as Butler suggests, additional performance is necessary—it is not enough to *be* thin. Further, because fat is socially and culturally constructed, rejection of fat identity through discourse is required for these authors to successfully claim a thin identity. As Leigh Gilmore puts it most succinctly, "Autobiography provokes fantasies of the real."[11] This intersectional act is reinforced in *Diet or Die* when Geyer asserts her agency as a wage earner when explaining her decision to join the sideshow to her brother even though she is subordinated as a fat woman. Although she has no obligation to consult with or seek permission from her brother, Albert, to work at all, when questioned in a pejorative manner about her prospective sideshow job, Geyer counters with, "I'm free, white, and over twenty-one."[12] Geyer asserts multiple subjectivities with this single phrase, which constructs the only identity categories that provide her with a sense of stable agency.

Memory, as invoked by the weight loss memoir, functions in a way that constantly reinforces the autobiographical subject as an oppressed and disenfranchised consumer. Geyer repeatedly writes about experiences as a producer and consumer of goods and services yet is denied full participation because of her size. As a teenager, Geyer took a job as a packer in a candy factory even though she was underage. She viewed employment as a viable alternative to school because of constant verbal abuse: "By this time even the teachers were calling me Fatso and other names." In an attempt to increase her earnings, Geyer transitioned to the Goldsmith Sporting Goods company a few months later and claims, "For the first time in my life I felt a feeling of accomplishment." By increasing her skill on the eyelet machine, the piecework nature of the position allowed for a substantial increase in wages. Though her disposable income increased, her purchasing power did not. "While most of the other girls spent their money for clothes and other accessories, I made regular trips to the bank and to the savings deposit window. I could not buy ready-made clothes, or high-heeled shoes, silk stockings or fancy underthings no matter how much I should have liked to do that, so I contented myself with my growing bank account."[13]

Geyer worked in several different factories and writes almost boastfully about her success at this type of work by earning at least double the 15-dollar-per-week base wage of her peers. "I was proud of my earning power and proud to tell everyone . . . Most of all I was proud of my bank account that rose almost as consistently as my weight."[14] Factory work acts almost as a metaphor for the space fat bodies are allowed to occupy as workers. So long as Geyer is anonymous and hidden, she can claim financial rewards. After repeated layoffs from the factories, Geyer attempts to find a different line of employment. A coworker suggests she learn a trade through stenography school as a means to more stable employment. Geyer has a sense of the discrimination she will face outside the factory and counters with, "What boss could give dictation with a 200-pound dolly on his knee?"[15] Certainly a number of troubling, gendered assumptions about employment are evident here as well. Geyer and a friend both apply to be switchboard operators and her friend is hired. Disappointed after not being hired despite possessing the same qualifications as her friend, Geyer then speaks with the personnel director who explains the reason for her rejection in a question masked as a declarative statement. "How could you possibly sit on our switchboard stools for a full day's work?"[16]

Geyer eventually finds some success pursuing a career as a manicurist. The relatively low cost of cosmetology courses compared to courses in other trades is a factor in her decision, but Geyer also considers the risk of finding a job after graduation as less than a clerical trade. "I knew placing me would not be easy, but I was willing to take a chance . . . even if I was not, in appearance, what the average beauty operator was."[17] Her initial placement allows for relocation to Miami working in a salon at a high-end hotel as a manicurist at the same rate as her most lucrative factory work. She befriends a wealthy shoe manufacturer in Miami who also contracts real estate and learns that one of his clients is the same factory superintendent that fired her from her last factory job. She convinces the shoe manufacturer not to conduct business with the man and helps negotiate a different land deal with the husband of one of her salon coworkers. Her shoe manufacturer friend, pleased with her assistance on the deal, gives her a $300 tip on his final nail-buffing appointment in Miami.

With the equivalent of five weeks' pay at her disposal, Geyer leaves her position at the salon to travel to Cuba for a vacation. She travels alone and is vulnerable to fat prejudice. Rather than a peaceful respite, Geyer sees employment as a solution to dealing with uncomfortable social encounters.

I was determined to have a wonderful time in this foreign playland. I soon learned that running away from myself, even to a strange land, was no answer; there was no escape. I was the same curiosity in Havana as I was in Cincinnati.

When I first checked into the hotel in Havana I was satisfied that my time here would be strictly vacation time. But when I left my room for any reason, when I walked through the lobby, when I went out on the street everyone stopped to stare and to laugh at me. Then I thought that I could avoid all of this uncomfortable experience if I were working in the beauty salon, hidden from public view.

Again, Geyer uses employment to retreat from what she considers public space. In Cuba, she is unable to find work in a salon, so she takes a position as a waitress instead. Unfortunately, the bar manager hires Geyer—the fat waitress—as a novel spectacle. Rather than endure mistreatment upon learning of the manager's true intention, she quits that position and returns home to Cincinnati.[18]

Even though Geyer writes to the weight-loss-as-salvation script when describing her pre-sideshow work, she also includes areas that claim agency. She earns wages as a worker, and despite being excluded from some areas of consumption as in finding ready-made clothes, shoes, and accessories in her size (which she considers the hallmark of full participation in femininity), she exercises power as a consumer of travel as described in the chapter entitled "New Scenes, Old Problem." Not only does she travel to Cuba intent on a vacation, but she also travels to California after quitting a job as a cosmetics demonstrator where her size prompts ridicule. On this trip, she meets a man "of as grotesque appearance as I."[19] This is the first time Geyer writes of meeting another fat person who is not a family member, albeit with initial scorn, and describes a pleasant encounter on the train. Alone after her companion departs in Montana, Geyer goes on to visit Yellowstone National Park, Seattle, San Francisco, El Paso, Juarez, Mexico, and St. Louis. In many of these places, she writes to the script again, recounting ways in which she was unable to fully participate in activities because of her size. At Yellowstone National Park, she takes a horseback tour, "and the next day practically everyone who was in the Yellowstone posse sought me out to tell me that the horse I rode died from overwork when they got him back to the stable."[20] In Seattle, she is ridiculed by theater ushers for needing accommodation after being unable to fit in the theater seat. Engaging in the confessional mode of diet discourse, Geyer describes these instances as evidence that her fat body is not fully functional in the world instead of highlighting discrimination. The confessional mode allows for recognition of discrimination only to the point that it becomes a personal call for transformation.

Working in the sideshow almost provides a glimmer of hope in Geyer's fat stigma narrative. Accepting Pearl Stanley's offer to join the Happy Land carnival sideshow in 1927 introduces Geyer to an alternate version of living as a fat woman in public space, but the sideshow version is not an innocent one. As explained by Stanley, "In this business you let yourself have fun while others see something funny in you. . . . You'll live a happy life in the show and you'll spread a lot of sunshine around while you make money."[21] Indeed, Geyer made more money in the sideshow than she did in any of her previous jobs, and her husband, Frank, lost his job in an automotive factory just before Geyer made her decision to join Happy Land. The agreement made with Stanley allowed for Frank to work as a general hired hand on the carnival, but this work earned less than half of what Geyer made, making her the primary income earner for the family. But her work was not without cost. The fat lady performance tropes relied on the same stereotypes and supported the same cruel treatment of fat people from which Geyer sought refuge. Also, fat ladies earned, on average, less than other sideshow freaks for their performance and relied on the sale of sexualized promotional photographs that included dressing in very short, low-cut, sleeveless baby doll dresses.[22]

Still, Geyer had some power over her career. She choose the stage name "Dolly Dimples," which created another layer of performance and separated real-life, miserable Celesta Geyer from her good-time, single glamour girl persona. As Geyer learned more about the sideshow industry, she distanced herself from Stanley and Happy Land for additional wages just as she did as a factory worker. From performance seasons 1927–38, Dolly Dimples performed with whichever carnival, circus, or fair that would pay the most money. At the height of her popularity during this period, she earned $100 per week in addition to wardrobe and travel expenses included in her contracts. During a brief performance on Coney Island, Dolly performed an act intended to be a parody of then "It Girl" Clara Bow as part of the "Wotta Fat Family."[23] Geyer describes this time in a mostly positive way, focusing on the camaraderie with other performers, the freedom she felt being able to eat as much and as often as she would like without ridicule, and the way clothes and furniture would be constructed without judgment to fit her. Material consumer conditions that should be available to all people regardless of size were available to fat women and men only if they were willing to become accomplices to the promotion of fat stigma. In this way, the sideshow becomes a site of protection. No longer socially isolated, Geyer and other performers begin to see their fat performance as sheltered from the oppression they once faced outside the show. Only upon reentering society as a "regular" fat person does the feeling of scorn return. Geyer describes returning to Cincinnati during a show break and being forced to endure the stares and remarks of a fat-hating public. "I did not like staying home, especially now, since the neighbors came by to look at me and see how big and fat I had grown. They laughed and laughed at Dolly Dimples who was now a pro in the fat business and I think they even took joy in seeing me for free."[24] In this passage, Geyer refers to herself as Dolly Dimples as she does in the title of the book, perhaps as a reminder of the separation between Dolly and Celesta. Though she is hurt by the staring and ridicule, Celesta-as-Dolly is a "pro in the fat business" and focuses on the economic impact of allowing a potential audience to see the show without paying rather than make the connection between her portrayal of Dolly and the real impact of the performance.

By 1950, Geyer had worked as a successful, professional sideshow fat lady Dolly Dimples for 23 consecutive seasons. The financial success of her career allowed for a custom-built home and furnishings:

> The design of my home including special structural features and custom-made furniture. The floors were all concrete slab, there were oversized doors, a wide shower stall and a king-sized johnny that was made to measure for me. The front- and rear-walk approaches to my home were big enough to accommodate both Frank and me, which allowed me the small pleasure of walking outdoors without crowding or being crowded off the walk. And I had an expansive drive to the front walk so I could be driven right to my front entrance.
>
> All of my furniture was luxuriously large and comfortable with concealed reinforcements. I had a wonderfully stuffed chair in the living room where I could sink into the depths of relaxation.[25]

For the first time in the memoir, Geyer describes material conditions required for living as a fat person outside the sideshow as simple facts rather than guilty admonishments or the punch line of a joke. Of course, according to compulsory diet discourse, this is the exact moment that a health scare attributed to fat would invite weight loss as the "deus ex machina" of "Before" body salvation.

Up to this point, I have specifically avoided the term "obesity." In keeping with fat studies principles, I have referred to people with large bodies as fat in accordance with the political project of reclaiming the term as a signifying descriptor.[26] "Obesity" or "obese" are nearly inescapable medical terms that pathologize fat bodies and contribute to discriminatory attitudes and practices. Because doctors categorize fat people as always already ill with an "obesity" diagnosis, receiving medical treatment can be a highly traumatic and discouraging experience. Fat patients in the United States are consumers of health care and often face the same barriers to access found in other consumer sectors with the addition of dismissive or hostile attitudes of medical personnel. Geyer faces all of these barriers when she experiences swollen ankles and shortness of breath in 1950. Initially, she does not interact with the doctor directly; her family serves as intermediaries and she does not find out the diagnosis of "a serious heart condition" until several days after her initial examination.[27] She "cannot" be undressed or put in a hospital bed and spends the night in a hardback chair sleeping in her street clothes. Without explicit explanation, both Geyer and her doctors assume that her condition is related to her weight, doctors are "somehow" able to complete the necessary diagnostic tests, and she receives treatment of metabolic dehydration and a limited diet of baby food. "For the next four days I was watched and treated like a six-months-old baby."[28] Finally, at the point of discharge, she is unable to be weighed because the hospital scales are rated for only 350 pounds. The moment of transformation begins with the doctor's advice: " 'Dolly, you have lived to diet; if you don't, you'll die. Think about it.' "

The narrative focuses on the change required of the ill individual rather than prejudicial discrepancies applied to fat bodies. Not three pages before, Geyer boasts about her "fully functional" home that has been specifically designed and constructed for her body. But in the hospital, she is subject to infantilizing treatment and left powerless by diagnostic and rehabilitative equipment that does not accommodate her, given an incomplete diagnosis based on body size, and denied food in a way that thin patients would not have to endure. Yet she believes the doctor's prognosis of death unless she pursues weight loss. In this moment, Geyer begins the eradication of her fat "Before" body with a strict 800 calories per day.

If the middle of the memoir begins to challenge the traditional weight loss memoir, the end safely returns the reader to the predictable script, which is nicely summarized in advice by Geyer's doctor as she is being released from the hospital:

> "You'll be out beyond the controls of the hospital and your doctor so you have to decide right now if you really want to continue to live. You can not go back to the kind of life you have known since you were a child. You certainly cannot look forward to working in circuses and carnivals as a side-show freak anymore. Rather you can look forward instead to becoming a normal beautiful woman—normal weight, normal appearance, normal activity in every way. You can look forward to living, doing, and enjoying everything a woman should."[29]

Geyer has been broken down to the level of infant and rebuilt in the image of a "champion" dieter. In the course of a year, Geyer loses 433 pounds and proudly proclaims that she is "deep in the habit of dieting and not eating."[30]

Despite a lengthy and diverse work history, extensive travel opportunities, and the creation of a home environment that accommodates her body in a comfortable way, by the end of the memoir Geyer declares that her life is better with an "After" body because she can fully participate in a consumer economy. As an "after," "it's a tremendous thrill to go to a movie, sit down in a regular seat and enjoy the picture like anyone else does," "it's a relief to buy a standard car," "it's a delight to hail a cab," and even "nice to go to the dentist now."[31] Finally, "gone are the days when the sight of me created mental havoc in the minds of innkeepers. Always when they saw my quarter-ton expanse they knew immediately that their beds and furniture were in for a beating and invariably they protected their investments with 'no vacancy' excuses and signs."[32] The fact that all of these opportunities would be available to her without changing her body if goods and services accommodated a wider range of body sizes is completely lost to serve the standard ending of a weight loss memoir.

At its worst, the weight loss memoir reinforces the misconception of willpower and control through dieting as the solution to prejudice, mistreatment, and barriers to material and economic access. Despite all the interesting travel and social experiences she encountered "before," the caption of an "After" photograph claims, "Present day Dolly can do anything, even have fun on the golf course." A second photograph shows Geyer trimming orange trees in her backyard.[33] A politically resistant reading of weight loss memoir acknowledges all the ways in which weight loss in response to fat stigma is flawed. Instead of viewing Geyer's weight loss as inspiring or triumphant, a resistant reading confronts it as unnecessary. Dolly Dimples "Before" lived a life that gave her the ability to pursue many interests, but the best Celesta Geyer can hope for "After" is a trip to the dentist and some yard work.

NOTES

1. Celesta Geyer and Sam Roen, *Diet or Die: The Dolly Dimples Weight Reducing Plan* (Hollywood, FL: F. Fell, 1968), 101.

2. Ibid., 102.

3. The text was also simultaneously issued by Chateau Publishing the same year with the title *The Greatest Diet in the World*, cribbing the Ringling Brothers Circus slogan, "Greatest Show on Earth." This version of the title would make sense only if the reader knew the slogan and its relevance to Geyer's work in the circus. This likely explains why *Diet or Die* is the more well known of the two versions.

4. Jane Nichols, " 'I Was a 555-Pound Freak': The Self, Freakery, and Sexuality in Celesta 'Dolly Dimples' Geyer's *Diet or Die*," *Journal of the Canadian Historical Association* 21, no. 2 (July 2010): 83–107.

5. Rosemarie Garland-Thomson, "Re-shaping, Re-thinking, Re-defining: Feminist Disability Studies," Barbara Waxman Fiduccia Papers on Women and Girls with Disabilities (Center for Women Policy Studies, September 2001), http://www.center womenpolicy.org/pdfs/DIS2.pdf.

6. Esther D. Rothblum and Sondra Solovay, eds., *The Fat Studies Reader* (New York: New York University Press, 2009), 2.

7. Hillel Schwartz, *Never Satisfied: A Cultural History of Diets, Fantasies and Fat* (New York: Anchor, 1990), 208.

8. Jean Nidetch, *The Story of Weight Watchers* (New York: W/W Twentyfirst Corporation, 1972), 204.

9. Rosemarie Garland-Thomson, *Extraordinary Bodies: Figuring Physical Disability in American Culture and Literature* (New York: Columbia University Press, 1997), 19.

10. Kathleen LeBesco, *Revolting Bodies? The Struggle to Redefine Fat Identity* (Amherst: University of Massachusetts Press, 2004), 4.

11. Leigh Gilmore, *Autobiographics: A Feminist Theory of Women's Self-Representation* (Ithaca, NY: Cornell University Press, 1994), 16.

12. Geyer and Roen, *Diet or Die*, 107.

13. Ibid., 45–46.

14. Ibid., 50.

15. Ibid., 45.

16. Ibid., 51.

17. Ibid., 52.

18. Ibid., 56.

19. Ibid., 58.

20. Ibid., 60.

21. Ibid., 112.

22. Nicholas, " 'I Was a 555-Pound Freak,' " 96.

23. Geyer and Roen, *Diet or Die*, 127.

24. Ibid., 128.

25. Ibid., 191–92.

26. Marilyn Wann, "Foreword," in Rothblum and Solovay, *The Fat Studies Reader*, xxi.

27. Geyer and Roen, *Diet or Die*, 192.

28. Ibid., 195.

29. Ibid., 199–200.

30. Ibid., 218.

31. Ibid., 222–23.

32. Ibid., 223.

33. Ibid., 225.

10

A Weighty Judgment: Reflections on Ethical Evaluation of Size

Rory E. Kraft Jr.

From reports that physicians are asking patients to zoos and veterinary offices in order to undergo X-rays and CT scans,[1] to the dismissive looks of passersby,[2] or "the lecture" from medical staff, it is all too common for society to judge those whose weight is above the cultural norm for beauty. Unfortunately, what I refer to as the "weighty judgment," or the judgment that one is lacking in moral worth based upon weight, is not confined to those who have not spent time considering the questions and problems of ethics. Recently, Daniel Callahan, who could safely be called a founding father of the discipline of medical ethics, claimed that perhaps shaming the overweight was the manner to go forward in producing a healthier society.[3]

What all of these judgments share is that the recipient of the judging (perhaps in some situations even the person making the judgment about him or herself) does not meet the societal standard for weight. This evaluation is commonly done not based upon a scale (though that can be the case), but is most often done by performing the "look test." One fails this test if she or he appears fat. "Failure" of this test often carries with it the failure of another test: a test for acceptability. Those in our society who fail the weighty judgment are considered to be lazy slobs who cannot or will not exercise self-control and are open to ridicule, hatred, or being ignored. What I find most interesting about these evaluations is that they are wrapped up in language that evokes discussion about someone's character, status as a person, or general goodness. These judgments are not just judgments about someone's weight; they are judgments about someone's moral worth.

In the following I examine first what standard approaches to ethics in the Western philosophical tradition have to say about judging others' moral worth. Following that I turn to medical ethics in particular to display the immorality of making a weighty judgment. Finally, I turn to the possibilities that a Health at Every Size (HAES) approach allows for appropriate moral considerations of the self and others.

A component in any discussion of the ethical considerations tied to weight must be the appropriateness of evaluating an individual on the basis of any given physical characteristic. These concerns have less to do with the medical appropriateness of a given protocol than with the moral appropriateness of considering an individual's moral worth or finding a moral failure to act in an acceptable fashion. The three dominant systems of ethics in the Western tradition are the deontological ethics of Immanuel Kant, the consequentalist ethics of John Stuart Mill, and the virtue ethics of Aristotle. Each of these approaches is briefly considered here

Kantian ethics is at its most simple a rule-based approach to ethics, where the rightness or wrongness of an action depends upon the type of action it is rather than the outcome of the action, the intent of the agent acting, or any other method that could be used to evaluate an action. The central method of analysis in his approach is a consideration of whether or not a potential action conforms to the Categorical Imperative, most easily understood as a test for whether an action can be universally applied without causing a contradiction.[4] Kant stated the Categorical Imperative in multiple different formulations; the formulation that is most applicable to the discussion of obesity ethics is the "means/ends" formulation, which requires that we each treat others always as an end in themselves, never merely as a means to an end.[5] This is widely accepted as being the source of our obligations to treat others with respect.

Kant's system of morality finds that we have a claim on the respect of other individuals and are "in turn bound to respect every other."[6] Acting in a contrary manner would be to give up one's own dignity, or at least to find acceptable and moral the abolition of self-esteem and dignity. While he acknowledges that it is perhaps impossible not to at times inwardly "look down on some in comparison to others ... the outward manifestation of this is, nevertheless an offense."[7] Further, even in the censure of vice one "must never break out into complete contempt and denial of any moral worth"[8] of another. Kant's system of ethics is a rule-based system, which does not allow for exceptions to moral duties. Thus under his system, we are each individually obligated to treat others with respect and never deny the moral worth of another.

Kant's brief discussion of gluttony is interesting in light of this discussion. While he holds that "stupefying oneself by the excessive use of food or drink" is a vice, the basis for this is "not the harm or bodily pain (diseases) that a human being brings on himself by it" but rather because he believes that there is a principle (though not a duty) for prudence.[9] Despite his comments on treating others with dignity, he states that gluttony "is even lower than the animal enjoyment of the senses, since it only lulls the senses into a passive condition."[10] He remains conflicted when it comes to the appropriateness of accepting an invitation to a banquet, which is "a formal invitation to excess in both food and drink," since there is a moral end at work in bringing "a number of people together for a long time to converse with one another."[11] Problematically, Kant sees gluttony as being a violation of duty to oneself through overindulgence, which carries a "physical harm ... which could perhaps be cured by a doctor."[12] Yet despite this view, he also holds that it is wrong to condemn others, and we cannot use Kantian tools to show that the evaluation of others (even those who fall short of contempt) is morally praiseworthy (or even acceptable). Kant thus gives us a mixed bag; evaluating others is arguably not morally right, yet evaluating oneself harshly may be.

The approach most commonly contrasted to Kant's ethics is a conseqentialist approach to ethics, which is closely associated with John Stuart Mill. Mill refined and updated a system of ethics from Jeremy Bentham and named this new system "utilitarianism." This system, unlike Kant's ethics, which focuses on individuals, emphasized the social connections between members of a community and a shared obligation we carry for others. In Mill's system of utilitarianism, the morally best action to take in any given instance is the one that will produce the greatest amount of happiness for the greatest number of individuals. The happiness to be considered in utilitarian theory is "not the agent's own happiness, but that of all concerned."[13] In contrast to a deontological approach like Kant's, Mill's consequentualism could potentially find that almost any given action is morally right, if that action results in more happiness for the whole than alternative actions. Yet even for Mill we can demand to be treated with respect and conversely others can demand that we treat them with respect. Failing to treat another in this manner is not just wrong, but an act of injustice. The practical problem here is that we often lose sight of the fact that we cannot obligate others to do as we wish. As Mill notes, there are things "which we wish that people should do, which we like or admire them for doing, perhaps dislike or despise them for not doing, but yet admit that they are not bound to do; it is not a case of moral obligation."[14] This is a practical problem for ethics because we need to realize that there are things that we would wish that others would do, but that our wishing of them to do so does not create an obligation on their part to follow through. These sorts of wishes seem to be at the bottom of many attempts by others to find that diminished moral worth accompanies increased weight. However, making this moral judgment is in itself an act of injustice and should be avoided.

Perhaps Utilitarianism provides us with more hope than Kant did. Where Kant left open the door for harshly evaluating oneself, Mill finds that happiness is the measure of all morality. It would be odd indeed if thinking harshly about oneself brought about increased happiness, so these critical self-evaluations are probably ethically wrong. In addition, the critical reflection of others' moral value seems to be clearly wrong in this schema. An additional possibility for utilitarian approaches is that the enjoyment that someone gets from preparing and consuming food not only counts as a moral benefit but also could establish that it is better for those who enjoy food to have a greater allocation of social resources.[15]

The third major approach in Western ethics is virtue ethics. This understanding is most closely associated with Aristotle and focuses less on the importance of individual actions (though they are considered) and more on a fully lived life. A central tenet of Aristotle's ethics is that the various excellences or virtues are understood to be the mean between the extremes of excess and deficiencies. This mean is not an arithmetic proportion true for all, but is an agent-relative mean. For example, just as we know that we need to feed Milo the wrestler more than a nonathlete, we know that we cannot set the marker between conflicting passions to an individual's specific mean derived from any set of individuals.[16] The virtuous action is one that is done "at the right times, with reference to the right objects, toward the right people, with the right aim, and in the right way."[17] Aristotle further believes that we come to find our own mean points by alternating between the extremes of excess and deficiency until we come to recognize the proper level of action.[18] Implicit here is that an intimate part of living the virtuous life will be reflection and evaluation of oneself. We each learn to live the good life by reflecting upon our past attempts, and through introspection come to see where we have fallen short of the mark or exceeded the appropriate level of acting.

When we consider Aristotle on the evaluation of others based upon weight, it appears that there are several pertinent aspects. First, as Aristotelian or virtue approach focuses on the complete life rather than on individual actions, it is clearly the case that individual acts that may raise the ire of others, such as the consumption of "nondiet" food in public, ought not be considered appropriate for ethical evaluation. We know not if the person eating an apparently sumptuous banquet has eaten anything at all that day, what his metabolic rate is, or any other aspect that may alter the appropriateness for consuming certain food types. Learning what to consume and how much to consume is something that occurs over time, first by erring to one extreme (too little food) and then the other (too much), until an agent comes to discover the amount and types of food that are proper for him. Secondly, Aristotle would hold that the proper understanding of what is appropriate needs to be done in light of the particulars of the situation. Individuals ought not be evaluated on the basis of their conformity to some arbitrary standard. Finally, we need to be aware of the fact that we really can evaluate someone only in light of a complete life. For self-evaluation, this means that we can see where we have been, our past mistakes and successes, and come to embrace the excellences that we potentially have. For evaluation of others, it means that it is highly inappropriate to dismiss someone as morally worthless because they fail to pass the "look" test for fitness.

If we turn from ethics as a general discipline to the specific area of medical ethics, we find both a continued usage of the theoretical approaches previously discussed and a set of new models developed specifically for use in medicine. Among these medical ethical theories is the dominant approach of principalism, which originates in the work of Thomas Beauchamp and James Childress. In their model, the principles of respect for autonomy, beneficence, nonmaleficence, and justice are to be key considerations in the analysis of a medical situation in order to determine the ethical action(s) to take.[19]

One of the standard concerns in medical ethics is an awareness of paternalism, which violates the principle of respect for autonomy. In medical paternalism medical practitioners, or the larger medical establishment, substitute their judgment about what are best practices for the patients' own judgments and beliefs. One manner in which paternalism is seen in the medicalization of obesity is in the standards that are used to determine which body mass index levels are considered overweight. These population analysis categories were revised in the United States in 1998 to correspond to World Health Organization standards, which resulted in approximately 25 million more Americans being overweight than had been the case prior to the change. As body mass index categories are widely used as a proxy for health status, this resulted in many more individuals being treated as ill. This is often seen in the discussion of weight and body mass index with patients going to a physician for a non-weight-related medical issue. The recent labeling of obesity as a disease by the American Medical Association seems likely to only make this medicalized judgment more pronounced.[20]

Another concern linked to Beauchamp and Childress's principle of respect for autonomy is ethical requirement for informed consent. Informed consent requires that an individual who is undergoing treatment understand the benefits and risks of that intervention as well as the underlying reasons for the therapeutic measure. To the extent that the uncertain link between health and weight is not discussed with patients, this ethical concern has already been violated. Further, when individuals are not given information on the failure to sustain weight loss (even assuming a causal link between weight and health) they are misinformed as to the possibilities of successfully treating their weight. An apt illustration of the problem of informed consent in weight management is to speculate as to how many individuals are informed that less than 15 percent of those who attempt a given medical intervention have long-term success from it.[21] If, as seems reasonable, we assume that few would attempt that intervention with full knowledge of the lack of success, we should question why weight loss regimens are so popular.

The principles of beneficence and nonmaleficence call for medical practitioners to do good and avoid harming others. Those who question the need for surgical interventions to treat weight are often drawing implicitly on these principles. Further, critics of these surgeries point out that the restriction or removal of portions of the digestive tract (in the words of Atul Gawande) "removes no disease, repairs no defect or injury."[22] As the issues surrounding the ethics of surgical intervention are complicated enough to require their own expanded discussion, I can do little more here than point to the links of those concerns to the failure to meet Beauchamp and Childress's principles.

The fourth principle, justice, is understood to be the source for concerns about resource allocation. Essentially, the distribution of goods or sharing of the burden of costs should be done in a manner that is just in order for it to be considered ethically good. In the consideration of weight issues, the amount of money that consumers spend annually in an attempt to lose weight (an estimate of between $30 billion and $50 billion was provided in a 1998 editorial in the *New England Journal of Medicine*) for the treatment of what has been labeled a global epidemic should raise ethical concerns.[23] Those who are considered ill are being faced with the bulk of the costs of treatment of that illness—despite public health campaigns that emphasize the community-based nature of the "causes" of overweight and obesity. As increased weight and lower economic class correlate strongly, this burden is coming disproportionately on those who would lack the financial resources to advocate for their treatment.

What this examination of Beauchamp and Childress displays is that the bulk of the activities that raise the ire of fat activists are those that the medical ethical establishment ought to find as not in keeping with the core principles of the profession. Put simply, medical ethical principles find that the weighty judgment and the corresponding medical activities that accompany it are not appropriate.

It is perhaps not surprising that the HAES approach to understanding weight is one that finds that the weighty judgment of the self or another is incorrect. At its core HAES calls for both self-respect and the care and concern of others. As Linda Bacon states, HAES calls for one to "shift your focus from hating yourself and fighting your body to learning to appreciate yourself, your body, and your life."[24] Since the focus of HAES is, by definition, not weight but health status, it becomes much harder to utilize a weighty judgment either on oneself or on another.[25] After all, it is tricky to look at another and tell if she is a marvelously skilled swimmer or if her cholesterol level is in a healthy range. Those sorts of judgments about health require not a "look test," which all too easily shifts into the dismissal of moral valuation, but instead either conversation or medical tests.

Perhaps one of the most visible assaults on weight as a replacement for moral worth comes from Marilyn Wann's "Yay! Scales," which display compliments rather than a numerical weight when one steps onto a scale. By calling for individuals to focus not on their weight but instead upon their self, Wann's scales provide a tangible manner to break free from being considered a number on a scale and instead seeing that one is a complete person. These scales also represent a physical manifestation of a larger fat-positive or fat acceptance movement.

The various perspectives and communities that make up the fat acceptance movement share a common feature in their dismissal of the appropriateness of the weighty judgment. These movements instead hold that fat individuals have been and continue to be considered of a lower class and social standing than those in the "normal" weight ranges. Their advocacy for equalized treatment in some instances includes moving for formal legal recognition (such as in the cities of Washington, DC, and San Francisco, California, and the state of Michigan). In other cases it takes the form of promotion of positive images of fat individuals in advertising, literature, and film. Yet across these approaches and communities, there is a central understanding that weight is not an indicator of moral failing(s).

When it comes to the weighty judgment, it seems clear that with the standard bearers of Western ethical theory, the evaluation of others as lacking in moral worth is itself a stance that is morally wrong. While there is some room for negative self-judgment, the three dominant modes all agree that it is not the place of an individual to make a weighty judgment. As weight is commonly linked in society to health, it is natural to turn to medical ethics to see how the weighty judgment fairs. By examining the principled approach of Beauchamp and Childress, we have seen that not only is the weighty judgment not proper, it also is the case that much of what occurs in a medical setting that could be construed as fat shaming apart from the weighty judgment is morally wrong. Finally, by turning to HAES and other fat-positive movements, we can see that at their base is the idea that judging another on the basis of her weight is a flawed proposition.

The weighty judgment, the idea that one can dismiss another's moral worth based upon the failure to pass a "look" test of appropriate size, is unfortunately pernicious. As shown, even while Kant held that it was inappropriate to judge another, he found it hard to pass up the appeal of the consideration of gluttony on another's part. There is something of finding another's perceived failures of self-control that can be all too empowering. Yet it is not as if watching, in shocked fascination, a special on cable television about an individual who has to be taken from an apartment through a newly created hole in the side of the building ought to bring greater feeling of self-worth. From the proliferation of such "health"/personality shows as Style Network's *Ruby* to the "weight loss competition" show *The Biggest Loser*, there is clearly a demand for watching the lives of "the other" who weighs in at some astounding figure. *The Biggest Loser* also allows the home audience to see the work that the contestants have to do in order to reform their lives—move into a group house, eat carefully monitored food (though there is often a "will test" to see if contestants can withhold from eating their favorite foods), and exercising for hours at a time while personal trainers chastise them for a lack of effort. These instances reinforce that the reason why "they" are fat is because "they" are lazy, make poor choices, and lack willpower. Yet this moral diminishment of others in the media can create a very real sense of self-loathing. Then the weighty judgment shifts from being about "them" to being about "me." As one begins to see herself as not worthy of moral treatment, then she is effectively dehumanizing herself and creating a situation wherein she acts as if she is not worth being treated well. This perhaps is one of the most jarring consequences of the weighty judgment: judging others and then oneself as not worthy of moral consideration brings one to the point finally of ceasing to find worth in one's own existence. But it is exactly that end point that we must see as the fatal flaw of the weighty judgment. Judging one in lacking in moral worth on the basis of size is itself a moral wrong and ought not be tolerated. Thankfully, the dominant methods of ethical analysis are in agreement on this point. Now the difficulty comes in getting action to follow through from theory.

NOTES

1. For an example, see Jenny Hope, " 'We Are Going to Have to Send You to the Zoo,' Doctors Tell Obese Patients Too Large to Fit in Hospital Scanners," *Daily Mail*, January 15, 2012.

2. See the "Wait Watchers" project by photographer Haley Morris-Cafiero.

3. Daniel Callahan, "Obesity: Chasing an Elusive Epidemic," *Hastings Center Report* 43, no. 1 (January–February 2013): 34–40.

4. Immanuel Kant, "Groundwork of the Metaphysics of Morals," [Grundlegund zur Metaphysik der Sitten] trans. M. Gregor, in *Practical Philosophy*, ed. M. Gregor (London: Cambridge University Press, 1785/1996), 37–108, 4: 402. (In keeping with scholarly tradition, this page reference is to the volume and page number in the German Academy edition of the complete works of Kant.)

5. Ibid., 4: 429.

6. Immanuel Kant, *The Metaphysics of Morals* [Die Metaphysik der Sitten], trans. M. Gregor, in *Practical Philosophy*, ed. M. Gregor (London: Cambridge University Press, 1797/1996), 353–603, 6: 462.

7. Ibid., 6: 463.

8. Ibid.

9. Ibid., 6: 427.

10. Ibid.

11. Ibid., 6: 428.

12. Ibid.

13. John Stuart Mill, *Utilitarianism* (Chicago: University of Chicago Press, 1906), 25.

14. Ibid., 73.

15. For more on this, commonly referred to as the Problem of Expensive Tastes, see R. Dworkin, "What Is Equality? Part 1: Equality of Welfare," *Philosophy and Public Affairs* 10, no. 3 (1981): 185–246.

16. Aristotle, *Nicomachean Ethics*, in *Complete Works of Aristotle*, ed. Jonathan Barnes, vol. 2 (Princeton, NJ: Princeton University Press, 1729–1867), 1106a36–b6. (In keeping with scholarly tradition, this page reference is to the Bekker page and line number, which derives from the 1831 edition of Aristotle's work compiled by Immanuel Bekker.)

17. Ibid., 1106b20-24.

18. Ibid., 1109b25.

19. Tom L. Beauchamp and James P. Childress, *Principles of Biomedical Ethics*, 6th ed. (New York: Oxford University Press, 2008).

20. American Medical Association, "AMA Adopts New Policies on Second Day of Voting at Annual Meeting," accessed June 20, 2013, http://www.ama-assn.org/ama/pub/news/news/2013/2013-06-18-new-ama-policies-annual-meeting.page.

21. For more on this statistic, see C. Ayyad and T. Andersen, "Long-Term Efficacy of Dietary Treatment of Obesity: A Systematic Review of Studies Published between 1931 and 1999," *Obesity Reviews: An Official Journal of the International Association for the Study of Obesity* 1, no. 2 (October 2000): 113–19.

22. Atul Gawande, "The Man Who Couldn't Stop Eating," in *Complications: A Surgeon's Note on an Imperfect Science* (New York: Picador, 2003), 162.

23. Jerome Kassirer and Marcia Angell, "Losing Weight—an Ill-Fated New Year's Resolution," *New England Journal of Medicine* 338, no. 1 (January 1, 1998): 52–54.

24. Linda Bacon, *Health at Every Size: The Surprising Truth about Your Weight* (Dallas, TX: BenBella Books, 2010), 1.

25. An in-depth discussion of HAES and its methods is beyond the scope of my work here. Instead I focus solely on the aspects that tie into (the lack of) the weighty judgment. For a larger examination of HAES, the best place to start is Linda Bacon's book.

11

How I Stopped Shoulding on Myself

Jessica Wilson

I was seated at a long table at a friend's weekly potluck. It was autumn of 2009 and I didn't know anyone else at the gathering, and I had made the risky choice to bring my new girlfriend with me. We were in Eugene, Oregon, a city that aspires to achieve the foodie credibility of Portland but with an added flair of activist and hyper-liberal roots. A lot of the food from the potluck came from guests' Community Supported Agriculture boxes, and meals were mostly vegetarian, if not vegan. As a newly registered dietitian, I sometimes struggled with declaring my profession in Eugene, since doing so often inspired a newly self-identified vegan, raw foodist, or locavore to proclaim and expound upon their eating manifesto for 60 minutes or more. We got settled with our food and began to eat when someone at the table asked about the latest book by a popular food writer. This book listed hundreds of rules that everyone should follow when eating or choosing food and the guest wondered what people thought about it. When no one spoke up with feedback the host mentioned I was a dietitian and might have something to say. Great, I thought, if this lasts an hour I will not win any awesome girlfriend points tonight. I started off with "Well, it is an interesting concept" while thinking of the least offensive way of saying that creating food rules that center around organic and locally grown produce, local seafood, and nothing that you cannot pronounce (because everyone knows how to say "quinoa" on the first try) is elitist and classist, not to mention a good way to make most of us feel guilty at some point, if not every day, for breaking the rules.

Right before my head exploded from the pressure, Mary, a family member of my friend, leaned in and said, "I don't know about you, but I went to Catholic school, and I've had enough of rules created by white, older men, if you know what I mean." Silence. My eyes locked with Mary's . . . and a halo of light appeared around her. Did that just happen? If it did, it was the most brilliant thing I had heard anyone say about the rash of entitled talking heads who have splashed onto the *foodscape* to tell all of America to put down that disgusting, conventional hamburger on a white bun and pick up that glorious, organic, leaner ostrich burger (bison if you can get it locally) but please add only lettuce and tomato from your garden or Community Supported Agriculture, pickles you canned last year, heirloom wheat buns from the local bakery, wild-harvested mushrooms, and mustard (no ketchup).

In Mary's comment and in the silence that befell the table, I recognized the magnitude of truth in her statement. We are members of American society, and our loudest and most lauded nutrition information providers are food writers, television "doctors," people who make a living shaming fat people to be smaller in unhealthy ways in the name of health (and TV ratings), and people writing and speaking about population or laboratory studies—all of whom have no idea what our individual bodies need. The people who entertain us and bring us the news now shape the way we view food and our health, and provide the ways to change both—they have successfully, and profitably, positioned themselves to be the experts on what we all need to be healthy. Additionally, computer programs have now become a stand-in, basing their advice on two to five simple data points like height, age, and weight. Each day brings another "Weird Food Trick," "Top 10," or "5 Foods . . ." for the way we should eat, contracting and contraindicating yesterday's advice. We have been told what we should be eating, how much we should eat, when we should eat, where we should buy our food, how we should cook our food, what we should never ever ever eat unless held at gunpoint (at the time of this writing it is processed carbohydrates), and of course to top it off we are told that our weight will tell us if we are properly following all of these *shoulds*. We are now *shoulding* all over ourselves with no way and no one to clean up the resulting mess.

Some of us are more inclined than others to adopt *right* versus *wrong* ways of thinking about food choices. I have had many clients come into my office for advice about healthy eating who say, "But I thought eating carbs/fat was bad for us . . ." The media, our peers, and some health professionals may reinforce black-and-white thinking about food and all-or-nothing views about what needs to be on our plate. Some people believe that fat-free foods and snacks portioned in 100-calorie packs are a "healthy choice" regardless of what they taste like or how they actually make us feel or affect our hunger. My clients have been told to believe, despite all evidence and experience, that sugar-free ice cream is healthy and tastes just as good as the original, that eating chalky protein bars for meals or snacks is a good choice since they are a "right food," and that counting calories, carbs, protein, or fiber is something they are obligated to do if they really care about their health. They've been told that their dessert choices are supposed to be healthy and come in preportioned, high-fiber, low-carb options right out of the freezer.

This messaging has resulted in a culture where some folks make food choices with nothing in mind other than body size outcomes like weight, size, and shape. This can be especially true for people who have been told that they need to lose weight at some point during their lives. I had this experience starting in childhood, through my adolescence, and even into adulthood. Labeled "overweight" as a child, before "childhood obesity" became a common phrase, I was told to eat less by medical professionals in order to be thinner. As an adolescent I was mocked for my size and I turned to food restriction as the solution.

In the pre-Internet '90s, my *shoulds* came from television commercials and "low-fat" messages. I used butter-flavored powder on dry toast (I do not recommend this), kept a public whiteboard tally of the calories I ate (or didn't eat), and chose highly processed, fat-free, preportioned food because I knew exactly how many calories were in them. I felt shameful about my eating habits and the pressure to change them accordingly to be thinner. In my early college years, I restricted food in order to avoid the "freshman 15," which resulted in weight loss and a rapid weight regain the same year. That opened the floodgates for feelings of failure, and knowing that if only I had followed my *shoulds* better, it wouldn't have happened. Trying to follow all of my *shoulds* exhausted me by my early twenties, and in my haste to do the "right" thing I had paid little, if any, attention to my well-being and quality of life.

Reflecting on those who now provide us with the *shoulds* in popular culture and online, I realized Mary was right; they tend to have a few things in common: most are white, most of them are older, many are men, and most are straight. I am none of these things. I'm a black, queer, early thirties woman. I can't think of anyone like me who is giving out food advice, and a quick Internet search affirms this. Among the key words I searched for ("black," "queer," "woman," "nutrition") tells me how important good *nutrition* is for *queer women*, and the *black* bean burger recipe Google provided does look delicious. In the twenty-first century, I am surprised that we are unable to recognize how the biological diversity that exists in our country could affect nutrient needs. I am not making the case that my differences give me radically different nutrient requirements for every food and nutrient than someone who is white, straight, and male, yet there are distinctions that, when compiled, become relevant to how I interpret messages received from health care providers and popular culture.

There are many reasons that one set of nutritional recommendations would not be appropriate for all people. To illustrate this I'll use myself as an example. The following are a couple of ways that make me different and how these influence the efficacy of the nutrition and food recommendations provided.

I AM BLACK

Vitamin D

When someone sees me they notice that I am black; I have darker skin than most of the people who make dietary recommendations. The darker someone's skin is, the less able they are to use the sun's rays to make vitamin D in the body.[1] If I look up guidelines for vitamin D on the U.S. Department of Agriculture's website, chapter 7 of the Dietary Reference Intakes tells me that "skin pigmentation" will affect vitamin D level.[2] Thankfully, I know that is a fancy term for lightness and darkness of skin color, but it does not say *how* vitamin levels are affected, and the rest of the 38-page document does not discuss specific recommendations for people with darker skin. The National Institutes of Health also tells me that people with darker skin have reduced ability to produce vitamin D from sunlight but stop there in addressing the issue, leaving out how these people need to alter their sun exposure or supplementation.[3] My body is different; if my primary source of vitamin D is through sun exposure, I am still unclear how much I need; is it more than the 5–30 minutes recommended?[4] By following the recommendations for the general population, I am not sure I will get what I need to be healthy and well.

My Ideal Weight?

I am also given messages about foods I *should* or *shouldn't* eat based on how I measure up to my "ideal weight range." This range is often calculated based on the "healthy weight" category of my body mass index (BMI), a ratio of height to weight. The equation, kilograms divided by meters squared, was developed by a statistician who found that he could predict a person's height given their weight, or weight when given their height, most of the time or for the *norm* of the population ... in the 1800s... in Belgium.[5] Not where I'm from, nor when I have lived. This equation had nothing to do with health in the 1800s, but in the twenty-first century it has become a primary motivator for people to change their eating habits to benefit their health. In the twentieth century, the experiment to determine that BMI was an effective way to label people was completed using men mostly in their forties and fifties— definitely not me.[6] Studies since the 1990s have demonstrated that blacks and other people of color are more likely to have a lower body fat percentage than white folk at the same BMI.[7] This means that my BMI, which I've been told is "good" or "bad" at different times in my life, and what I *should* do differently to fix it (eat less), is an invalid measurement for me. Thankfully, I know now that neither my BMI nor my size has anything to do with whether I am healthy or at risk for chronic diseases, but by the time I learned this there were years of negative messaging about food, calories, and weight that had built up in my mind. Again, these are more reasons that listening to someone else's advice about what I need to be healthy has not served me well, and will not do so in the future.

I AM QUEER

My queerness, or lack thereof, does not directly impact my nutrient needs or that of my community. It does impact the standards of beauty to which we are held. Many messages directed toward women about eating have more to do with achieving a smaller size rather than health and well-being. Some queer women may choose to be larger in stark contrast to society's praise of smaller and smaller women. My female queer community is more accepting of different body shapes and sizes, and appreciates this diversity. Most of us know that difference in size is simply difference and not inherently *bad* or *good*. We do not spend time discussing our beach bodies or lack thereof; we show up at the beach. We do not have discussions about health in direct relation to size. I feel affirmed in this community, regardless of my size. In this community, mainstream nutrition recommendations for ways women can reduce their size do not apply.

As my needs are different from the norm, so are others'. I do not expect healthy people from different cultures and countries than my own to (a) be eating the same foods, (b) be the same size, or (c) have the same biochemical and anthropometric markers seen in tests as those in the United States. I also do not expect everyone in the United States, a lovely combination of many cultures, to be labeled as healthy or unhealthy, and worthy or unworthy based on invalid measures and collective *shoulds*. Eating is very personal for each one of us and rather intimate too; the food we eat literally becomes us. Right now we have one general set of guidelines for all people telling us what we should become.

There are people in the media, pharmaceutical companies, and medical providers who create and share food and health recommendations assuming that everyone's needs are the same. Computer programs and apps for mobile devices provide caloric recommendations after gathering two data points. Nutrition research completed using a specific segment of the population is often extrapolated to everyone, often with a commentator's position that if it is good for one person, it will be great for everyone. Our federal government has provided the same nutritional recommendations for every person divided only by sex, age, pregnancy, and lactation.

I do not think that the one-size-fits-all approach to health has helped to make our nation happier, healthier, or better able to make food choices. It certainly did not help me recognize and appreciate the nourishing capacities of food at an early age, nor provide me the ability to treat my body well. When we heed food advice from a computer, popular culture, or a human who has not personalized the advice nor incorporated our individual identities, experiences, and behaviors, we will not get advice that is relevant to us. There is great diversity in this nation: sex, race, size, class, ability, ethnicity, and country of origin to name just a few. With this great diversity, it would make sense that there would be diversity in food needs as well. We are constantly making food choices—what, where, when, etc.—and there needs to be a better way to do so.

It is time to do things differently and value our own ability to guide our food choices above others'. It is time to shake off the *shoulds* and begin to let our individual bodies tell us what they need. This is not an easy task, but I have found the principles of mindfulness to be helpful when figuring out my needs and I am honored to introduce them to you.

Mindfulness has roots in Buddhist tradition, but the principles are not tied to religion. When we are mindful we remain in the present moment and do not stay attached to thoughts about the past or future. Mindful eating is being present while eating, making food choices, and listening to your body. It incorporates your attention to cues, awareness of your senses, and noticing responses. There is not a rule to follow or a list of boxes to check off when eating mindfully; it is an ongoing process and we refine it with practice. Eating mindfully is not something that can be done perfectly, and this gives us permission to give up our right/wrong thinking and rules. Mindful eating happens without conscious restraint and while unattached to distant outcomes like weight, size, or shape, and is in stark contrast to messages that affront us daily. To eat mindfully, one must work on letting all of these messages go.

Awareness and nonjudgment are two principles of mindfulness. Awareness is the constant practice of noticing all of your body's senses and responses in the present moment. To be *aware* is to observe everything that goes on within us and around us when eating. This includes the feelings that we arrived with, the responses we have to our food, and how these may change moment to moment. At first it may be uncomfortable to become more aware of your body, its cues and responses. It may be especially difficult for those of us who have worked hard to undue our bodies' natural cues and not notice feelings about food. And with practice we can become better aware.

Creating an environment that minimizes distractions when first practicing awareness may be helpful. A space dedicated only for eating and not working, relaxing, or playtime may improve the ability to be aware of the experience. This may be a cleared space at the table, a counter, or even a blanket or placemat that gets rolled out on the floor at each meal. When working on this in grad school I dedicated a corner of my table to be clear from work at all times, which helped me clear my mind while eating. Creating a physical space for awareness sets a good intention to be mindful. Decide if eating without the television, radio, or computer on will be best for paying attention to your meal, and if attending to a ringing or buzzing phone while eating will help you practice. By dedicating time and space to awareness of the experience, the subtle cues that have remained hidden from attention may become more noticeable.

If you take a few seconds to reflect upon your typical evening meal, what comes to mind? Possibly it is the food itself, but it may also be the television show you typically watch at that time, the radio program you listen to, the mealtime company, the stress of decision making, the balancing act to get food on the table, or the rush in order to slide into your dinner chair in time to eat with the family. These are some of the thoughts and feelings that we may bring to our meals without realizing we've done so. For me the thoughts of what to do *after* dinner are already distracting me before I sit down to eat my meal. These subconscious thoughts and stressors influence our ability to be aware of our eating. As we notice what we bring with us to our meals, we can work on letting these go before eating our food. It doesn't have to take long; would taking three deep breaths be helpful, or reading a calming quote posted on the fridge do the trick? I like to draw my shoulders up to my ears and drop them while exhaling to center myself. Just as we would prepare for something else that needs full concentration, we can prepare for a meal with the same level of intention in order to be fully present. The more we practice the less we will need to prepare. While eating and working on becoming more aware, there will inevitably be thoughts that drift in that are related to the future or past, and that is okay. We can work on observing these thoughts without becoming attached to them, and know that if they are important, they will return after our meal.

As the journey continues, awareness of the other things that exist during the eating experience may increase. The sights, smells, sounds, and textures of food may magnify when your awareness is heightened. Each of these senses may impact responses to food differently. There may be more attention to one over the other, or one sense may be more important to feelings of satisfaction. At the beginning of a mindfulness practice, checking in with your feelings and how you're responding to food can be helpful. You can ask yourself, "What else did I bring to the eating space today?" or "How have my feelings changed as I continue to eat?" or "What do I most notice about this meal, and which senses are not as prominent?" After the meal the ways that foods affect the body will continue to evolve within us and we can notice how food affects the day. We can notice how it settles in the body, if we feel energy enhanced or depleted after eating, and how long that food sustains satisfaction.

Awareness also includes attention to hunger, satisfaction, and fullness. For those of us with typically developed endocrine and digestive systems, we were born with a natural ability to regulate our eating via hunger, satiety, and full-ness cues. We may be able to recall watching a baby or child eat their food and how easy it was for them to begin and stop eating according to how much food they needed. Those cues may have become muddled as we have aged if not attended to. This may be especially true for those of us who have ever inten-tionally restricted food. Instead of listening to these cues, various forms of restraint may guide the beginning, end, and size of a meal.

Most people are clear about the concept of hunger and what it feels like. We often discuss only its extremes: "I'm starving right now," or "I'm so hungry I could eat a horse!" Yet there are varying degrees of hunger as well as more than one type of hunger. We have both physiological and what I call psycho-logical hunger, which involves all of the other ways that we can be motivated to eat food. When practicing mindfulness we may be better able to notice the difference between the two. You may notice that physiological hunger comes on gradually, starting at a low level and gaining in intensity.[8] This type of hunger is our body signaling that it is time to find more food. Psychological hunger can come very intensely and may lead to cravings for certain foods.[9] There are many senses and feelings that can influence psychological hunger, including emotions, environments, sights, smells, and our mouth.[10] To deci-pher between the two you can observe how quickly your desire to eat came on, and whether or not you need to eat specific foods to be satisfied.

Satiety, or satisfaction, is less discussed in the United States, and being satisfied after eating remains more of an elusive topic in our culture. I often describe satiety as the body signaling that it has had enough nourishment for that moment. When beginning to notice this signal, observe how your hunger level changes as you eat, and at different points you can check in with, "Does my body need any more food right now?" When the answer is "no" you may be satisfied. If this answer is unclear at first, have compassion for yourself and continue to practice with the same intention.

Different foods contribute to satiety in different ways, and by cultivating awareness you will be able to notice this and choose foods according to what your body needs at the time. As your ability to notice improves, you will become more aware of the various other feelings that occur with satiety. This concept can be tricky for those who don't feel satisfied unless their plate is empty or until they are physically full, or for those who feel like they should be satisfied after eating a certain amount. Satisfaction was particularly difficult for me to conceptualize. Before I began learning about mindfulness I felt like I had never been full at meals, and I could always eat more. In fact I had been *full* many times before, but because I was used to eating with restraint, I was never truly *satisfied* at meals. I was used to eating according to a rule or restraint and did not know what to tune into between hungry and full. I was shocked at my ability to develop my cues again and eat in accordance.

To practice noticing your cues, asking yourself questions may be helpful. You can check in with, "Am I experiencing physiological hunger or a different type of hunger?" or "How are my hunger and satiety cues evolving moment by moment?" "Why do I not go back for more food even though I am still physiologically hungry?" or "Why am I continuing to eat though my body does not desire more food?" By staying present when eating and noticing body cues and responses, you will be better able to rely on your body as a guide to what it needs.

The other important component to mindful eating is withholding judgment, from both our food choices and ourselves. For those of us who have been told we *should* eat this or *shouldn't* eat that to change our size, shape, or weight, this may be especially hard. This concept even goes against the marketing that judges the food for us, telling us that it is *Guilt free!* These thoughts and resulting feelings about food can be hard to undo, and take time and practice. Eating a *bad* or *good* food may result in feelings of guilt or pride. Negatively judging a food choice may lead to more mindless and emotional food choices since the day is "ruined." Withholding judgment will keep us present and prevent us from focusing on the distant outcomes of that food choice. In mindful eating, the feelings that we observe are those that we experience as a direct response from eating the food, not from judging it. When we refrain from judging food we are able to let our bodies feel our experience, integrate it, and learn from it. To decide whether you are judging foods positively or negatively, check in to see if certain foods make you feel like you have won or lost after eating them. Notice whether food choices are based on whether or not you *should* eat it, rather than the food's ability to nourish you or meet your need in that moment.

Principles of awareness and withholding judgment can be applied to emotional eating, or eating in response to psychological hunger, not physiological hunger. Sometimes when we eat in response to how we are feeling or reacting to life, our awareness comes at the end of the moment in phrases like, "How did I eat that whole ice cream/pizza/cake?" or "I feel horrible after eating all of that." And judgment may follow—"I shouldn't have eaten all of that" or "That was a really dumb idea" or "I need to stop my emotional/stress eating." When practicing mindfulness you have the opportunity to notice whether you are psychologically or physiologically hungry. If not physiologically hungry, you can decide whether or not to eat food to satisfy the hunger. And if the choice is yes, you can maintain your awareness while eating and eat until you are satisfied. Afterward you can notice how the food feels in your body, and go on with the next moment of your life. You may also choose to eat past satiety and the same principles would apply. It is not *wrong* to eat more food than satisfies the body, and when you eat mindfully you are aware and are making the conscious choice to do so. You have not tuned out the body's cues entirely with the intention to avoid noticing. By remaining in the present, awareness of the food's effects in the body is maintained. Eating in response to psychological hunger or eating past satiety is neither bad nor wrong, though it is wise to pay attention to whether eating in response to psychological hunger becomes a pattern or increases in frequency. This may be a sign that something in your life is out of balance and addressing it may lead to improved well-being.

Both principles also apply to social settings. Social events like dinner or potlucks may be avoided if someone has already eaten "too much" food or "too many" calories. They may also undernourish the beginning of their day by restricting food in order to earn "permission" to overeat at an event. Instead of trusting the body to signal satisfaction in these situations, people may choose to miss out on social interactions in the former example or set themselves up to be overly hungry and disengage from the body's natural cues in the latter. Each of these situations can be different by becoming aware of satisfaction cues and enjoying the event. By withholding judgment, there will not be thoughts that cloud concentration and take away engagement in the moment. With awareness and removing judgment, we are able to choose to eat and not eat foods provided while keeping a clear mind and staying present.

When you are aware and remove judgment you become the keeper of what your body needs and desires in order to be healthy and happy. You are then the expert. You do not count, portion, or restrain yourself; you rely on your body to tell you what it needs and when. I do think that Mary was right; I too have had enough of *shoulds*, rules, and restraint, and hopefully you have too. I have found that undoing the years of negative messaging about food, size, and weight has been one of the hardest tasks I have undertaken, and well worth the effort. I invite you to join me on the path of mindful eating, and to welcome the freedom that you have had all along to make your own food choices. This will be your own journey, and you will never arrive at an end point. The goal is to continually notice. While on this journey display compassion toward yourself, as you would to anyone else learning a new skill. There are likely years of messaging and restraint to undo.

NOTES

1. "Dietary Supplement Fact Sheet: Vitamin D," Office of Dietary Supplements, National Institutes of Health, last modified June 24, 2011, http://ods.od.nih.gov/factsheets/VitaminD-HealthProfessional/#en2.

2. "Vitamin D," Dietary Reference Intakes, http://www.nal.usda.gov/fnic/DRI/DRI_Calcium/250-287.pdf.

3. Garabed Eknoyan, "Adolphe Quetlet (1796–1874)—the Average Man and Indices of Obesity," *Nephrology Dialysis Transplant* 23, no. 1 (January 2008), doi: 10.1093/ndt/gfm517.

4. Ancel Keys et al., "Indices of Relative Weight and Obesity," *Journal of Chronic Diseases* 25 (1972): 329 –43, http://web.mit.edu/vincenta/www/BMI/indices_of _relative_weight_and_obesity.pdf.

5. Eknoyan, "Adolphe Quetlet (1796–1874)."

6. Keys et al., "Indices of Relative Weight and Obesity."

7. P. Deurenberg, M. Yap, and W. A. van Stavern, "Body Mass Index and Percent Body Fat: A Meta Analysis among Different Ethnic Groups," *International Journal of Obesity* 22 (1998): 1164–71, http://www.nature.com/ijo/journal/v22/n12/pdf/ 0800741a.pdf; Sarah M. Camhi et al., "The Relationship of Waist Circumference and BMI to Visceral, Subcutaneous, and Total Body Fat: Sex and Race Differences," *Obesity* 19, no. 2 (2011): 402–8.

8. Megette Flecher, "Different Types of Hunger," The Center for Mindful Eating, Teleconference Handout, March 23, 2010, http://www.thecenterformindfuleating .org/Resources/Documents/ADifferentTypesofHungerHandout.pdf.

9. Ibid.

10. Jane Chozen Bays, *Mindful Eating: A Guide to Rediscovering a Healthy and Joyful Relationship with Food* (Boston: Shambhala, 2009).

12

Thin Fat Activism

Moniqa Paullet

You will be happy if you stay thin.
Make sure you don't put on weight.
You'll be richer if you're thin.
You'll spend your whole life battling your weight.

These are the messages told me every time I visited certain family members growing up. They were persistent enough that I internalized them. I spent 25 years swallowing, dwelling on, and obsessing over the knowledge that I would spend the entirety of my life—DECADES—battling my weight, battling my genes, a waging war against my weak and traitorous body. I blamed my family for their weight and my seemingly inevitable fate alongside them as if being fat were the worst thing that could happen to a person—worse than death—because everyone "knows" it is.

Racism, sexism, and homophobia are weeded out and discouraged on a large scale, through federal and state legislation and the high social costs incurred by alienating others; however, fat shaming has somehow held out as a bastion of not only publicly accepted but even lauded and medically promoted discrimination, though the research overwhelmingly shows that obesity is only a body size, neither a disease nor indicative of individual health, moral failing, or personal worth. A society that values individuality, the pursuit of happiness, and personal autonomy cannot also suffer bigotry and discrimination.

The so-called obesity epidemic is largely overblown. Rates of obesity among women have held steady for at least a decade.[1] And possibly longer, but the definition of "overweight" body mass index was arbitrarily altered in 1998, magically transforming 35 million Americans into an "unhealthy" weight literally overnight. Why the change? "Eight of the nine members of the National Institutes of Health task force on prevention and treatment of obesity have ties to the weight-loss industry, either as consultants to pharmaceutical companies, recipients of research money from them, or advisers to for-profit groups," the *Newark Star-Ledger* reported.[2] Whatever the purported reasons, those responsible for determining the definition of health in America stood to profit financially if there were more "unhealthy" people, never mind that body mass index measures neither body fat nor any indicator of actual health and wellness.

A disease by definition is a condition that impairs normal functioning. Body size alone does not fit that definition, and treating obesity as a disease leads to misdiagnosis in MORE THAN 70 million people. "Psychologist Deb Burgard examined the costs of overlooking the normal weight people who need treatment and over-treating the obese people who do not. She found that BMI profiling overlooks 16.3 million 'normal weight' individuals who are not healthy and identifies 55.4 million overweight and obese people who are not ill as being in need of treatment," according to Linda Bacon.[3] Sick people go untreated and well people are given prescriptions. Fully one-third of obese people are not at risk for diabetes and heart disease, and one-quarter of normal-weight people are at risk.[4]

In addition to ignoring the ailments of thin people, the practice of treating obesity as a disease effectively discourages overweight people from seeking medical treatment, and those who do find difficulty in even obtaining treatment. Weight loss is regularly prescribed for everything from strep throat to infertility to stubbed toes.[5]

While obesity may show a higher correlation with diabetes and heart disease, so does living under constant stress, such as being stigmatized and shamed for one's body size, as discovered by researcher Peter Muenig.[6] Though it's been repeated ad infinitum, *correlation is not causation* seems to be a hard concept for many to grasp. What it means is that researchers have found a relationship between higher weight and having a greater chance of being afflicted with certain diseases. But correlational studies do not indicate whether one causes the other, or whether one or both may be caused by or related to a third factor. Muenig further mentions, "Statistical models suggest that the desire to lose weight is an important driver of weight-related morbidity when BMI is held constant." So the stress of ill-treatment may be to blame in whole or in part for "obesity-related diseases."

Combined with overall lower mortality rates for overweight persons than normal- and underweight people,[7] does it still make sense to assume that body fat causes illness rather than living with the daily stresses of size-based discrimination and body shaming?

Though nearly 70 percent of the U.S. population is overweight or obese,[8] fat acceptance is a critical social movement to improve the quality of life for thin people as well. Consider the $66 billion weight loss industry,[9] the prevalence of eating disorders, and the lack of positive body image among women.

A survey by Dove found that a mere 2 percent of women think they are beautiful, from among thousands across the globe.[10] With the so-called obesity epidemic making headlines, the very real issues of eating disorders, size discrimination, and body shaming take a backseat to the fabricated problem of size itself.

Millions of men, women, and children devote their energies to worrying and obsessing about their weight and food instead of pursuing activities that bring them joy and appreciating foods that add mental, emotional, and social value to life. If people's ambitions revolve around controlling the size of their bodies, how many trillions of hours are devoted to restriction, with children missing out on enjoying birthday treats, and men and women spending more time and effort on calorie counting than on creative endeavors and technological advances?

This is more than a thought experiment based on personal perceptions:

- 46 percent of 9- to 11-year-olds are "sometimes" or "very often" on diets, and 82 percent of their families are "sometimes" or "very often" on diets.
- 51 percent of 9- and 10-year-old girls feel better about themselves if they are on a diet.
- 42 percent of first through third grade girls want to be thinner.
- 81 percent of 10-year-olds are afraid of being fat.
- 80 percent of all children have been on a diet by the time that they have reached the fourth grade.[11]

Two-dimensional statistics from an article tell little. Picture the children you know—yours, your friends', your nieces, and even you at that age worrying about dieting and fatness when the biggest concerns ought to be skinned knees and decorating the right size poster board for class projects. The pervasiveness of diet culture psychologically harms children, effectively indoctrinating them to accept a lifetime of media-driven and culturally normalized shame, discrimination, and self-hatred.

I keenly remember feeling my first instance of body shame in the sixth grade when we were first required to dress for gym class in uniform T-shirts and cotton shorts. All the other 11-year-old girls had skinny little legs, but I had soft, fleshy thighs. I self-consciously lifted them from the ground when sitting cross-legged so that they wouldn't flatten and spread so wide. And I'd look around at all the other girls with their skinny-minny legs and wonder why mine were so big. I was 11 and as average as can be, active in soccer and dance classes several days a week. And I felt bad about my body for looking different because I somehow believed I was supposed to be (or try to be) the same as the other girls.

I learned to be ashamed to show my thighs—in shorts or skirts or swimsuits—because I had more than bones and skin or because I dared to show my body, dared to fail to be acceptably decorative to the world as defined by the media ideal. And I was never an overweight child. My story isn't special and it isn't okay. It isn't unique and that is even worse. Every word from the mouths of grownups about being good or being bad for eating certain foods and comments praising appearance teaches children that food is valuable only for calories and people are valuable only when they're conventionally attractive.

Appearance-based discrimination is problematic because it is based on mistaken assumptions about the value of weight loss and one's ability to attain and maintain it, and on fallacious conclusions about individuals' health, morality, willpower, and inherent value.

If increasing public health is the desired goal, then encouraging healthy behaviors and improving access to health services, a variety of foods, and enjoyable movement and exercise options will achieve that goal. Research repeatedly shows that increasing healthy behaviors improves health, as measured by blood pressure, cholesterol, glucose levels, and similar physiological indicators, regardless of a person's size or whether any weight is lost. A study from 2012 found that "when stratified into normal weight, overweight, and obese groups, all groups benefited from the adoption of healthy habits, with the greatest benefit seen within the obese group."[12]

These findings are not all new, and there has long been evidence to support a shift in focus from weight loss to the adoption of healthy behaviors. A study from 1986 found that "with or without consideration of hypertension, cigarette smoking, extremes or gains in body weight, or early parental death, alumni mortality rates were significantly lower among the physically active."[13]

As an alternative to weight loss efforts, Health at Every Size (HAES) is a paradigm shift that recommends behaviors for improving overall health instead of assuming weight loss as a panacea for all that ails. Its basic tenets are:

- To focus on improving health physically, mentally, and emotionally
- Respecting diversity of bodies and appreciating one's own, regardless of size
- Mindful eating based on internal cues of hunger, satiety, and appetite of a variety of foods that improve feelings of well-being
- Finding movement one enjoys doing for its myriad benefits independent of weight loss, gain, or maintenance
- Ending weight bias and discrimination

HAES values the practice and implementation of evidence-based medicine and research over the default "everybody knows fat = death" ideas perpetuated by the media, health care practitioners, and society at large. Normal eating bears no resemblance to any kind of intentional dieting or restriction, or how many people treat food and calorie tracking.

I gave up calorie counting after college because it made me a neurotic, obsessive, cranky, and miserable person. It does that to a lot of people, and it qualifies as disordered eating, falling far outside the parameters of health. I was one of the *lucky* few who could easily manipulate my weight through exercise alone and I enjoyed doing it. Weight loss has always come easily for me; maintenance has not. For most of my adult life, my weight has fluctuated wildly within a 20-pound range, which, for a long time, I believed was normal. While it's normal in that it aligns with nearly everyone's experiences with weight loss and regain, but it is not healthy or natural. The single most common long-term outcome of dieting is weight gain, typically leading to weight cycling, which does more harm than being heavy.[14]

> Normal eating includes the ingestion of healthy foods, the intake of a mixed and balanced diet that contains enough nutrients and calories to meet the body's needs, and a positive attitude about food (no labeling of foods as "good" or "bad," "healthy" or "fattening," which can lead to feelings of guilt and anxiety). Normal eating is related not only to health maintenance, but also to acceptable social behavior, and is both flexible and pleasurable.[15]

A reported 35 percent of "normal dieters" progress to pathological dieting. Of those, 20 to 25 percent progress to partial- or full-syndrome eating disorders.[16] And yet "health care" providers continue to recommend weight loss to patients entrusted to their care, a practice that is more harmful than healthful to people across the board.

Beyond calorie counting, I quit all other forms of restricted eating after learning about the all-too-common cycle of food restriction consistently triggering a binge response, guilt, and repeated attempts at restriction. The concepts of permission and intuitive eating allow me to eat better overall and enjoy every minute of it. Detractors argue that intuitive eating encourages people to give up on health and stuff their faces at daily all-you-can-eat buffets. This is a straw-man argument based on nothing ever proposed or practiced by real-life proponents of HAES. The purpose of eating is to feel well, and nobody feels good stuffed to bursting at every meal. Having a healthy relationship with food means appreciating not only its nutritional value but its emotional, social, cultural, and comfort values too and trusting your body to normalize fluctuations, such as partaking wholly of a holiday feast with loved ones, or becoming distracted and missing a meal entirely.

Even those who would argue that health is an important and worthy goal must admit that, based on the research, intentional weight loss efforts are the very definition of unhealthy and long-term weight loss is impossible for all but a tiny fraction of those who attempt it. Study after study bears this out, and commercial diet peddlers are legally required to clearly advertise that their products don't work for most people with "Results not typical" labels ever present in the fine print.

> Attempts to lose weight typically result in weight cycling, and such attempts are more common among obese individuals. Weight cycling results in increased inflammation, which in turn is known to increase risk for many obesity-associated diseases. Other potential mechanisms by which weight cycling contributes to morbidity include hypertension, insulin resistance and dyslipidemia. Research also indicates that weight fluctuation is associated with poorer cardiovascular outcomes and increased mortality risk. Weight cycling can account for all of the excess mortality associated with obesity in both the Framingham Heart Study and the National Health and Nutrition Examination Survey (NHANES). It may be, therefore, that the association between weight and health risk can be better attributed to weight cycling than adiposity itself.[17]

I support HAES because I'm a skeptic and my life depends on evidence-based medicine. There is no research that supports intentional weight loss as a healthy behavior. "That weight loss will improve health over the long-term for obese people is, in fact, an untested hypothesis. One reason the hypothesis is untested is because no methods have proven to reduce weight long-term for a significant number of people."[18]

Next time you or someone near you makes comments that moralize food or bodies or dieting, consider stopping them. It matters. Diet talk invites more diet talk, and self-criticizing does the same. So consider interrupting that talk and expressing a desire to avoid engaging in or listening to people making degrading comments about those you care for, including themselves. If you wouldn't stand for a stranger on the street calling a friend or coworker a cow for accepting a slice of birthday cake, why let anyone say the same about herself? We're in this together and no one can survive it alone.

Dr. Linda Bacon authored a peer-reviewed article[19] that compiles information from numerous studies that support the fact that intentional weight loss is detrimental to health, as well as supporting the HAES approach:

> Concern has arisen that this weight focused paradigm is not only ineffective at producing thinner, healthier bodies, but also damaging, contributing to food and body preoccupation, repeated cycles of weight loss and regain, distraction from other personal health goals and wider

health determinants, reduced self-esteem, eating disorders, other health decrement, and weight stigmatization and discrimination.

And in addition:

Only studies with an explicit focus on size acceptance were included. Evidence from these six RCTs indicates that a HAES approach is associated with statistically and clinically relevant improvements in physiological measures (e.g., blood pressure, blood lipids), health behaviors (e.g., physical activity, eating disorder pathology) and psychosocial outcomes (e.g., mood, self-esteem, body image). All studies indicate significant improvements in psychological and behavioral outcomes; improvements in self-esteem and eating behaviors were particularly noteworthy.

Pursuit of health and fitness is not a moral or social obligation. If someone wants to paint pretty pictures all day every day because that is what brings joy and meaning to her life, then that is her right. Widely prescribed, 150 minutes of moderate physical activity per week is perceived as a magical number—the answer to life, the universe, everything—and certainly key to prolonging life and banishing death and disease, which are inherently impossible and preposterous notions for humankind. Social proscriptions for fitness sound increasingly like an Orwellian future society's mandates.

Whereas health was once defined as the absence of disease, public health initiatives have morphed to promote the pursuance of the greatest possible physical fitness and longevity, failing to account for issues of dis/ablism and access to reasonably priced quality foods and safe, enjoyable movement options. Dis/ablism refers to prejudices and discrimination against people with disability, injury, mobility restrictions, etc. It is impossible for some people to exercise, but weight loss interventions fail to acknowledge this. Furthermore, gym memberships are an expensive luxury, and safe neighborhoods for outdoor movement aren't a given in every community. Higher rates of obesity are found among impoverished populations in the United States, presumably because accessing a variety of good-quality foods is expensive compared to calorie-dense "junk food,"[20] in addition to the costs of accessing fitness facilities.

The Centers for Disease Control and myriad other professional organizations recommend at least 150 minutes of moderate-intensity aerobic exercise PLUS two days of strength training per week for adults. This has been touted widely in the media as an easy way to guarantee fitness and health, a magical number, but, considering again issues of poverty and access, many find themselves without the time.

"Moderate-intensity" exercise includes options such as walking at three miles per hour, water aerobics, slow bicycling, and gardening, activities that many people don't "count" as exercise. Have I been failing bare minimum recommendations because I mostly do *only* "vigorous-intensity" types of movement? I should be elated because this knowledge makes "Perfect Fitness" more attainable, right? But it makes me angry that this definition was never made clear and that there are so many other people who are alienated and feel themselves failures because they think they can't meet these standards.

Fitness is not a moral imperative or societal obligation. It's important, so I'm saying it twice. Obesity is not a major cause of the rising costs of health care. Advancements that lead to greater longevity allow more people to get sick without dying and cost billions in health care. "Per capita spending on health care for adults would rise by 65 percent—from $4,550 in 2007 to $7,500 in 2020, CBO [Congressional Budget Office] estimates—largely as a result of the continuation of underlying trends in health care that have led to rapidly increasing spending for all adults regardless of weight."[21]

Fitness, movement, and exercise are personal choices. Independence and the right to pursue happiness are pretty damn important. Self-autonomy is pretty damn important. You can choose to do what you want to do. You do not have to do things that make you miserable or because you hate your body and yourself. Very few people succeed at hating themselves thinner or healthier.

While the recommendations for 150 minutes are based on good research, it's also true that any small amount of exercise can impart mental, emotional, and physical benefits. It's also important to note that the research suggests that you don't have to do the workout all at once. I choose to go all out for 10 to 15 minutes a day in a high-intensity, mixed cardio and body weight workout composed of squats, jumps, and pushup variations. It's a more efficient use of my time.

What works for one person will not work for every person. I'm young and healthy with a base level of fitness to draw upon from childhood gymnastics, dance, soccer, and color guard, so I can't preach about how easy it is to find enjoyable exercise without sounding like a privileged, dismissive jackass. (Admitting it is the first step.) And I'd be lying if I did. Sticking with the exercise bandwagon can prove to be far more difficult than it sounds; falling off the bandwagon at one point or another is inevitable, and for many of us: frequent.

There will always be people invested in reaping unearned advantages from the seeds sowed by oppression. It's much easier than actually trying to be a good person, cultivate talents, or do anything productive with their lives. Let them think their "hard work" spent chasing after thin privilege is the same as working hard to overcome prejudice, or raise a family, or pursue greater or higher knowledge, or survive in the face of challenges. It's easier to pant on a treadmill and think yourself better than someone else than actually do something that makes you a better person, friend, partner, or member of the community.

— Arte to Life, founder of This is Thin Privilege tumblr

The thought of casually reaping the benefits of being white, straight-sized, middle-class, and conventionally attractive while ignoring what my friends and family suffer because of it sickens me. I am well aware of the concept of privilege and I try to recognize my thin privilege and white privilege, the privileges of being able-bodied, conventionally attractive and cisgender, middle-class and a university graduate, and so on. These privileges allow me to practice HAES without being questioned for my food and fitness choices. They allow me to afford the food and fitness of my choice (my favorite running shoes and an adequately supportive sports bra don't come cheap). They allow me to speak about HAES without being judged a failure at dieting. They allow me to debate without my appearance being called into question as a motivating factor in my activism. They afford me the time to read, write, and comment and the opportunity to read research beyond what the fear-mongering media interprets as best-selling. It allows me to sidestep uncomfortable disagreements about the necessity of dieting for weight loss because my enthusiasm for fitness absolves me of the need to count calories.

I cannot refuse these unearned benefits of privilege, but I can learn to use them to help others by challenging the status quo. Acknowledging that a culture of fat shaming harms everyone of every size is a step toward working together to change that culture. Having allies strengthens a movement.

I'm a thin fat activist because I'm a feminist. Because even I've been a victim of size bigotry and appearance policing and the commodification of women's bodies as public property open to unasked-for public use, judgment, and scorn (e.g., street harassment). I have been the victim of body shaming and mocking and direct insults from strangers and from family. I was told flat-out last year by a brand-new doctor who asked nothing of my food and exercise habits to lose weight. I had just run three miles that morning and was devastated. I fired her.

As a skeptic, I am appalled at the cultural myths about the benefits of thinness and the conflation of weight with health. As a humanist, I am appalled at the rampant casual concern trolling and discrimination against fat people.

As a human I am so tired of hearing everyone, especially people I care for, spew hate about their bodies and their weight, and I am constantly saddened to see the submission to the lie that thin is the same as happy and healthy, and that a specific body size is good and valuable and desirable.

Changing the situation for marginalized groups will garner benefits for all of society. Instead of expecting people to change their appearance or to spend every waking moment working to stay slim in order to avoid stigma and shame, promoting acceptance of all body types will eliminate the stresses that correlate with disease and increased mortality. Recognizing people's value and worth independent of their appearance widens the talent pool in every field and creates myriad opportunities for progress and innovation.

One person can influence and educate a wide social network through word and action. One person can shut down diet talk and body shaming in his presence. One person can model body positivity and encourage her friends to do the same through social media. One comment dissenting from false assumptions about weight and health can act as a ray of light to the downtrodden reader and can plant a seed to grow in a skeptic's mind.

I wasn't a fat ally from birth, nor are most; I'm a convert and not the only one. Activism works; it has helped me and thousands of others discover the truth about weight and health, privilege and unjust discrimination. I cannot undo the hateful and ill-informed opinions I espoused in the past, but I can write, teach, debate, and practice, focusing on the value of individuals as humans, self-worth as separate from beauty, beauty as separate from body size, and options to pursue health and body acceptance.

Acceptance doesn't come easily; it takes practice. It takes a long time to unlearn the harmful programming society and family have given us about beauty, weight, health, and personal obligation to pursue and maintain them. It takes patience and perseverance, repetition until you can internalize and believe that you can be happy and healthy and fulfilled at any size. Life won't wait on weight loss, and we have only one life to enjoy; don't waste it accepting self-hate and shame, or any external hatred either.

People are valuable because they are human, not because they look a certain way. And everyone deserves a fair chance to pursue happiness without being discriminated against, daily insulted and trolled, and widely shamed for their appearance.

NOTES

1. John Wihbey, "U.S. Obesity Trends and Neighborhood Effects," *Journalist's Resource*, Harvard Shorenstein Center, January 5, 2012, http://journalistsresource .org/studies/society/medicine/u-s-obesity-trends-neighborhood-effects#

2. The Center for Consumer Freedom, *An Epidemic of Obesity Myths* (Washington, DC: Center for Consumer Freedom, 2005), http://www.obesitymyths.com/downloads/ ObesityMyths.pdf.

3. Lucy Aphramore and Linda Bacon, "Weight Science: Evaluating the Evidence for a Paradigm Shift," *Nutrition Journal* 10, no. 9 (2011), doi: 10.1186/1475-2891-10-9.

4. Daniel J. DeNoon, "Obese and Healthy," WebMD.com, (2008), http://www .webmd.com/diet/news/20080811/benign-obesity-malign-normal-weight.

5. "First, Do No Harm: Real Stories of Fat Prejudice in Health Care," http://fathealth.wordpress.com/.

6. Peter Muenig, "The Body Politic: The Relationship between Stigma and Obesity-Related Disease," http://www.biomedcentral.com/1471-2458/8/128.

7. K. M. Flegal et al., "Excess Deaths Associated with Underweight, Overweight, and Obesity," *Journal of the American Medical Association* 293, no. 15 (2005): 1861–67.

8. Centers for Disease Control, http://www.cdc.gov/nchs/fastats/overwt.htm.

9. John LaRosa, "U.S. Weight Loss Market Forecast to Hit $66 Billion in 2013," http://www.prweb.com/releases/2012/12/prweb10278281.htm.

10. http://www.prnewswire.com/news-releases/only-two-percent-of-women -describe-themselves-as-beautiful-73980552.html, 2004.

11. http://www.ndsu.edu/fileadmin/counseling/Eating_Disorder_Statistics.pdf.

12. http://www.jabfm.org/content/25/1/9.abstract?etoc.

13. Ralph S. Paffenbarger Jr., et al., "Physical Activity, All-Cause Mortality, and Longevity of College Alumni," *The New England Journal of Medicine*, 314 (1986): 605–13, doi: 10.1056/NEJM198603063141003.

14. Aphramore and Bacon, "Weight Science."

15. Raquel Franzini Pereira and Marle Alvarenga, "Disordered Eating: Identifying, Treating, Preventing, and Differentiating It from Eating Disorders," *Diabetes Spectrum* 20, no. 3 (July 2007), http://spectrum.diabetesjournals.org/content/20/3/141.full.

16. http://www.ndsu.edu/fileadmin/counseling/Eating_Disorder_Statistics.pdf.

17. Aphramore and Bacon, "Weight Science."

18. Ibid.

19. Ibid.

20. http://ajcn.nutrition.org/content/79/1/6.full.

21. How Does Obesity in Adults Affect Spending on Healthcare?, September 8, 2010, http://www.cbo.gov/publication/21772.

13

Come Out Come Out Wherever You Are: Queering a Fat Identity

Julianne Wotasik

For as long as I can remember I have been fat. I was a fat child, a fat teenager, and a fat adult. I do not recall any moment in my life where I did not identify as fat. It has been my primary identity and has influenced my life and my choices more significantly than my gender, race, and religious identities. Long before I embraced it, being fat has been something I could never escape and could never, even for a moment, hide.

I have a lot of social privilege as a queer person: I present as feminine and pass as straight. Very few people would guess at my queer identity unless they are specifically told. This identity is one I could have chosen and can choose to hide. Among those currently in their thirties, the average age of "coming out" is 21.[1] That is accurate in my case. I came out as queer to my friends and family in my early twenties.

My coming out as queer coincided with another coming out. Obviously, everyone who saw me knew that I was fat. When I came to a place of self-acceptance and came to see my fatness as something to celebrate rather than something to try to change, I realized that I needed to come out, not just as obviously fat, but as proud of being fat. As Abigail Saguy and Anna Ward put it, "Specifically, the hypervisibility of fat changes what it means to come out as a fat person, compared to what it means to come out as gay or lesbian."[2]

I have found that when we, as fat people, are seen as apologetic of our size, and seen as trying to change our size, we are given a sort of approval. We are judged as imperfect but, people say, at least we are working to improve. The idea of a fat person not trying to change their size is shocking and appalling to many people. It is hard for many people to conceptualize how a fat person could genuinely like their body and not wish it were thinner. Coming out as proud of a body that doesn't meet society's expectations opens one up to oppression and shaming even beyond that of simply being fat. Saguy explains:

> Fat activists regularly describe the experience of coming out as fat and choosing to no longer pass as "on-the-way-to thin" ... coming out as fat involves a person who is easily recognized as fat affirming to herself and others her fatness as a nonnegotiable aspect of self, rather than as a temporary state to be remedied through weight loss.[3]

Queer oppression still exists and is enacted every day. That said, we've seen a steady improvement in the general public acceptance of queer people. For instance, we've seen growing approval of same-sex marriage. "The rise in support for same-sex marriage over the past decade is among the largest changes in opinion on any policy issue over this time period."[4] Sadly, this trend is not repeated among fat people.

Harriet Brown discusses how, in a time of public acceptance and tolerance of differences, the stigma of being obese may be at an all-time high:

> Public attitudes about fat have never been more judgmental; stigmatizing fat people has become not just acceptable but, in some circles, de rigueur. I've sat in meetings with colleagues who wouldn't dream of disparaging anyone's color, sex, economic status or general attractiveness, yet feel free to comment witheringly on a person's weight.[5]

With public disapproval of fatness so high, just existing as a fat person is difficult. Coming out as someone who celebrates body diversity, including fatness, has been a challenging journey for me.

When I came out as queer to my friends and family, some were disapproving but most were accepting of my queer identity. Many of my straight friends were very supportive of my coming out. The only opposition I received was due to the religious beliefs of some of my family. When I came out, and as I continue to come out, as fat celebrating I have often been surprised at who is the most disapproving. While I have never experienced another queer person's disapproval of my queer identity, I have had a number of other fat people disapprove of my stance as fat celebrating.

I think that the queer rights movement has made some specific progress that the fat acceptance movement has yet to achieve. The queer rights movement has done a great job of helping the general public understand their message that queerness is not a choice. I also believe that queer activists have successfully spread the message that there is nothing wrong, harmful, or deviant about being queer. Lastly, I think that the queer community has been effective in helping queer people understand that they are acceptable, just as they are, and that they are deserving of equal rights and fair treatment.

More and more people are agreeing that queerness is not a choice. Most scientists and psychologists today agree that, although we can choose whether to act on our feelings, sexual orientation is not a conscious choice that can be voluntarily changed.[6] If you accept that people cannot choose to be either gay or straight, it seems logical to conclude that people should not be treated unequally based on their sexual orientation.

It can be argued that it is just as scientifically evident that fat people cannot change their size as it is that queer people cannot change their orientation.[7] Unfortunately, regardless of the scientific research, public opinion continues to insist that body size is a choice and is entirely within our control. Even medical providers—people who are supposed to treat patients based on medical science—place fault for body size on fat people's shoulders. Doctors often assert that body size is about personal responsibility and utilize stigma and shame as if they are health care interventions.[8] With the general societal consensus being that fatness is a choice, despite scientific evidence, the logical leap to treating people equally, regardless of weight, is not even attempted. Studies show that when people believe something is innate, not chosen, they show more tolerance.[9]

The belief that fatness is somehow a choice, that there exists a possibility of manipulating one's weight, not only contributes to the general public opinion about fatness but also affects the way fat people deal with their own fatness. If it were more widely understood and accepted that fatness is not a choice and cannot be successfully manipulated, more fat people would be likely to fight the stigma they experience and join the ranks of the fat acceptance movement.

Earlier in 2013 Exodus, a large organization founded to help gay people "change" into straight people, closed its doors—apologizing publicly for their work.[10] This would be the equivalent of Weight Watchers closing its doors and apologizing for all of the harm it caused the millions of people who have paid them money and trusted the information they disseminated. Exodus admitted that it failed gay people by suggesting that they could (or should) change their sexual orientation. If Weight Watchers were to admit that it has failed fat people by suggesting they could (or should) change their size, I think it would mark incredible progress in helping the general public to understand that fatness is not a choice. People used to think that "praying away the gay" worked because queerness was inherently immoral—a view that I experienced then about my queerness and that I experience now about my fatness.

Is it enough to understand that queerness, or fatness, is not a choice? The queer rights movement has gone further, successfully spreading the message that there is nothing wrong, harmful, or deviant about being queer. Certainly, there are still people who would disagree, but those people are fewer and fewer.

Religious groups in the United States, especially Christian churches, have been a huge source of resistance to accepting queer people. For at least several centuries, Christian churches have staunchly maintained that homosexuality is a sin and they have shunned gay people. "In the five years since the LDS church sent busloads of the faithful to California to canvass neighborhoods, and contributed more than $20 million via its members to support [Prop 8], it has all but dropped the rope in the public policy tug of war over marriage equality."[11] The Mormons have backed down from their fight against marriage equality. While they haven't opened their churches to queer people, or declared that homosexuality is not a sin, many other churches have done just that. One of the first churches established for queer people was the Liberal Catholic Church, in Sydney, Australia, in 1916.[12] Now, just under a hundred years later, if you visit www.gaychurch.org (the largest gay-affirming Christian Church directory in the world), you'll find almost 7,500 entries of gay-affirming churches and congregations.

Sadly, fatness is far more villainized now than 100 years ago. The fat rights movement has yet to successfully spread the message that there is nothing wrong, harmful, or deviant about being fat. "The war on obesity" has been waging for several years. "[Fat people] are made monsters—blamed by shocking shoddy research for everything from workplace costs, to healthcare costs, to fuel usage; unwilling combatants in a war by which the government seeks our eradication, preyed upon by a $60 Billion industry that sells snake oil in the promise of weight loss that will cure our social stigma by working the wrong end of the problem."[13]

My personal experience has certainly been that most people feel that being fat is synonymous with being lazy, overeating, and even being sinful. I have heard fatness condemned from church pulpits, from the White House, on sitcoms, and in conversation with peers. My fatness has been used as a reason for my doctors to lecture me, even though they admit that weight loss attempts almost always fail. My fatness has been justification for family members to decide that I "don't take care of myself," even when they don't actually know about my self-care or habits. I have been judged, criticized, and mocked because so many people are convinced that fatness is wrong—something that must be changed and avoided. They see fatness as harmful—leading to certain health issues—and deviant, a sure sign of laziness and gluttony.

It is not just thin people who have this opinion of fatness; my experience has been that many fat people agree with the prevailing negative beliefs about them. The fat acceptance movement has a long way to go in helping fat people understand that they are acceptable, just as they are, and that they are deserving of equal rights and fair treatment whether they want to change their body size or not.

I have been a part of the queer rights movement for almost as long as I have been a part of the fat acceptance movement. From my observation, the queer community has a much stronger presence. From rainbow flags, to subsets of neighborhoods that are known for their gay populations, the queer community is easy to locate. In 2012, it was reported that the Human Rights Campaign—the largest queer rights organization—had more than 1.5 million members.[14]

Having a visible community not only makes the queer rights movement more powerful when it comes to spreading messages and influencing legislation, but it provides support for queer people. It is not hard to find support groups for dealing with a myriad of queer-related issues, from coming out to queer relationships to dealing with discrimination. There are LGBT community centers in every major city in the United States, providing counseling, support, and community for queer people. One online LGBT calendar lists more than 200 gay pride parades and events over the next year,[15] some of them involving more than 400,000 people.[16]

It is not hard to see why having this large, loud, proud community has been helpful in proving support for queer people. Of course there are many queer people still struggling with their queer identity and internalized homophobia, but there are millions of proud, confident queer people in this country alone. I would not be surprised if the majority of these proud queer people credited their queer community as at least part of what helped them get to where they are in their journey of self-acceptance.

It is hard to embrace self-acceptance when you feel isolated and alone. I, personally, credit the fat acceptance community for much of my progress toward self-acceptance. If I had never become involved with people who believed in celebrating size diversity, I don't think I would have been able to embrace myself or see the beauty in people of all sizes.

Unfortunately, the fat acceptance movement doesn't have the healthy, growing community that the queer rights movement has developed. Founded in 1969 (the same year as the Stonewall riots), the National Association for the Advancement of Size Acceptance is the oldest fat acceptance organization in the United States but has only a few hundred members currently.[17] There are certainly pockets of fat acceptance community, and I am lucky enough to have found one of them in Los Angeles, but our community is not in the millions like the queer rights movement. These figures are upside down when you consider that it is estimated that almost 70 percent of adult Americans are fat,[18] whereas as few as 3.5 percent of adult Americans are queer.[19]

The fact that the fat acceptance movement is not grounded in cohesive social groups with their own practices, values, and culture is, we would argue, the reason why the movement has not yet developed a strong counter-culture and why coming out as fat is more about rejecting negative stereotypes than about affirming group practices, beliefs, or values. Wann speaks to this when she says that "fat people have yet to find a point of anger that would mean no turning back. Fat people still go along with blaming ourselves—rather than blaming the prejudice against us—when we're treated as second-class or untouchable."[20]

It is hard to fight for rights you don't believe you deserve. Perhaps the most essential thing that the fat acceptance movement needs is to help fat people understand that they are acceptable, just as they are—then they will believe that they are deserving of equal rights and fair treatment. Ragen Chastain, a prominent voice in the fat acceptance community, writes, "The first step, the very first step, is that fat people need to decide that they deserve respectful treatment and then demand it."[21] Chastain's blog is followed by more than 8,000 people and has received more than 3 million hits. Her work and the work of other activists has created an online community that is growing. Perhaps fat acceptance will find its community and empowerment through the Internet in the way that the queer rights movement has found it in social groups, neighborhoods, pride events, and in-person organizations.

Coming out as fat celebrating has been a challenge for me at times—it opens me up to further stigma as a fat person because I dare to be proud of my fatness. But I will continue to come out as often as possible because it serves my community and me. Harvey Milk, a queer activist who is a hero of mine, said:

Every gay person must come out. As difficult as it is, you must tell your immediate family. You must tell your relatives. You must tell your friends if indeed they are your friends. You must tell the people you work with. You must tell the people in the stores you shop in. Once they realize that we are indeed their children, that we are indeed everywhere, every myth, every lie, every innuendo will be destroyed once and all.

I like to think that this is true, not only of coming out as queer, but of coming out as someone who chooses to celebrate size diversity rather than despise it. The world is full of beautiful people—I want everyone to see that, so I'll continue to work up the courage to come out as queer, as fat, and as determined to help change society's narrow ideals.

NOTES

1. Rachel Williams, "People Coming Out as Gay at Younger Age, Research Shows," *Guardian*, November 15, 2010, accessed December 28, 2013, http://www.theguardian .com/world/2010/nov/15/gay-people-coming-out-younger-age.

2. Abigail Saguy and Anna Ward, "Coming Out as Fat: Rethinking Stigma," *American Sociological Association Social Psychology Quarterly*, accessed December 28, 2013, http://www.sscnet.ucla.edu/soc/faculty/saguy/ComingOutasFat.pdf.

3. Ibid.

4. Pew Research Center, "Growing Support for Gay Marriage: Changed Minds and Changing Demographics," Center for the People & the Press, March 20, 2013, accessed December 28, 2013, http://www.people-press.org/2013/03/20/growing -support-for-gay-marriage-changed-minds-and-changing-demographics/.

5. Karen Barrow, "The Stigma of Being 'Fat,'" *New York Times*, March 15, 2010, accessed December 28, 2013, http://well.blogs.nytimes.com/2010/03/15/the-stigma -of-being-fat/?_r=0.

6. Natalie Timoshin, "Sexual 'Conversion'? American Psychological Association Says Not through Psychotherapy," *Psychiatric Times*, accessed December 28, 2013, http://www.psychiatrictimes.com/articles/sexual-%E2%80%9Cconversion%E2%80 %9D-american-psychological-association-says-not-through-psychotherapy.

7. T. Mann and A. J. Tomiyama et al., "Medicare's Search for Effective Obesity Treatments: Diets Are Not the Answer." *Am Psychol.* 62, no. 3 (2007): 220–33.

8. Harriet Brown, "For Obese People, Prejudice in Plain Sight," *New York Times*, March 16, 2010, accessed December 28, 2013, http://www.nytimes.com/2010/03/16/ health/16essa.html.

9. Christian Crandall and Rebecca Martinez, "Culture, Ideology, and Antifat Attitudes," *Personality and Social Psychology Bulletin* 22, no. 11 (1996): 1165–76.

10. David Sessions, "Exodus Closes, Marking Official End of the Ex-Gay Movement," *Daily Beast*, June 21, 2013, accessed December 28, 2013, http://www .thedailybeast.com/articles/2013/06/21/exodus-closes-marking-official-end-of-the-ex -gay-movement.html.

11. Stephanie Mencimer, "Mormon Church Abandons Its Crusade against Gay Marriage," *Mother Jones*, April 12, 2013, accessed December 29, 2013, http://www .motherjones.com/politics/2013/04/prop-8-mormons-gay-marriage-shift.

12. Jeffery P. Dennis, "Gay and Lesbian Churches and Synagogues," *gbltq*[T], p. 1, accessed December 29, 2013, http://www.glbtq.com/social-sciences/gay_lesbian _churches.html.

13. Ragen Chastain, "Fatty Was Here and Still Is," *Dances with Fat* (blog), June 6, 2010, accessed December 29, 2013, http://danceswithfat.wordpress.com/2013/06/10/ fatty-was-here-and-still-is/.

14. "The HRC Story," Human Rights Campaign, accessed December 29, 2013, http://www.hrc.org/the-hrc-story/about-us.

15. http://www.nighttours.com/gaypride/, accessed December 29, 2013.

16. "LA PRIDE 2013 Brings Large & Diverse Crowds," LA Pride!, accessed December 29, 2013, http://lapride.org/news/news_article.php?id_art=56.

17. "About Us," National Association for the Advancement of Size Acceptance, accessed December 29, 2013, http://www.naafaonline.com/dev2/about/index.html.

18. "Health, United States, 2012," U.S. Department of Health and Human Services, p. 33, accessed December 28, 2013, http://www.cdc.gov/nchs/data/hus/ hus12.pdf#063.

19. Gary J. Gates, *How Many People Are Lesbian, Gay, Bisexual, and Transgender?*, The Williams Institute, April 2011, accessed December 29, 2013, http://williamsinstitute.law.ucla.edu/wp-content/uploads/Gates-How-Many-People-LGBT-Apr-2011.pdf.

20. Abigail Saguy and Anna Ward, "Coming Out as Fat: Rethinking Stigma," *Social Psychology Quarterly* 74, no. 1 (2011): 53–75.

21. Ragen Chastain, "Casualties in the War on Obesity," *Dances with Fat* (blog), accessed December 29, 2013, http://danceswithfat.wordpress.com/2011/11/19/casualties-in-the-war-on-obesity/.

14

Women of Color in Size Acceptance Activism

Irene McCalphin and Juana Tango

When we were initially asked to expand upon the topic of why there is a need for women of color (WOC) leaders in the fat activist movement, both of us viscerally expressed the internal knowledge, "Duh, isn't it blatantly obvious?" But then we reflected upon our actual experiences in the world at large, in communities resisting oppression, and specifically in the interactions we've both had within the fat activist movement. What we immediately concluded was equally clear: that which is obvious to WOC is quite likely to remain unseen to folks who do not have firsthand experience living in a fat WOC's body.

A fat activist movement that doesn't incorporate WOC leadership will not comprehend nor acknowledge our experiences, may inadvertently or intentionally not address the marginalizations fat WOC are subjected to based on the intersectionality of our identities, and by rendering our experiences invisible such a movement will ultimately fail in its goal of creating a world accessible for *all* fat people. The fat activist movement must include WOC leadership, because our knowledge and experience are key to successfully achieving a world where everybody has just access to opportunities and resources.

Resistance to sizeism by fat women of color is by definition a movement that draws upon intersectional marginalizations. It is, therefore, impossible to discuss such a topic without addressing all of those experiences. Additionally, both the authors believe that in order to truly eradicate social systems of oppression, the intersectionality of all resistance movements must be incorporated into rendering all oppressions obsolete. A just world cannot exist unless all citizens have access to justice. Therefore, while our focus in this chapter is primarily fat WOC activists, it is vital to note that ultimately the successful eradication of sizeism must further include the knowledge of fat people who experience the gamut of intersectionalities including disability, sexual orientation, class, age, and transgender and nonbinary gender oppressions. Until that is achieved we all will continue to reside in a socioeconomic system of subjugation.

Drawing upon the experiences of other social justice movements for a brief moment, let's consider how successful two of these movements have been at eradicating the oppression they're focused on addressing. Imagine if the feminist movement was comprised only of men. Would women have obtained the right to vote or own property or have access to education in such a movement? Or was it only when the human beings being subjected to the oppression became the activists to end it that feminism became a movement? Would feminism exist without women? In the United States, first and second wave feminism primarily centered on the experiences of white women. Those first feminist waves managed to increase access to some social-economic institutions, but they did not succeed at dismantling the sandy beach of sexism. As the third wave of feminism began to address the experiences of WOC, greater strides toward more accessible access have widened opportunities not only for WOC but also for white women. One need only look at the ratio of male to female salary to see the results. In 1963 women made 58 cents for every dollar earned by a man.[1] In 2011 women earned 82 cents per male dollar. While African American women and Latinas still earn significantly less than white women, addressing the inequalities of pay that includes the intersectionality of racism has resulted in a closing of the gender gap pay inequality. If WOC earned what white women earn, the disparity would diminish even further. In other words all women benefit when the marginalizations WOC are subjected to are part of the feminist/womanist resistance to sexism. As fat WOC, we authors cannot begin to experience a humane world without addressing sexism.

Indulge us while we briefly stray to incorporate commentary on another movement. When sexual and gender identity social justice movements first began in the United States, the first voices to be acknowledged were gay men, closely followed by lesbian rights groups. Would gay men have had the understanding, passion, or commitment to address the ways heterosexism impacts women? What about the experiences of transgender people? Would cisgender folks queer or straight address the inhumane treatment of nonbinary human beings? Each time another letter is added to the acronym GLBTQIA (gay, lesbian, transgender, queer, intersex, asexual), it is added because the experiences of folks who identify as being represented by that acronym character were rendered invisible, because the socioeconomic oppressions were not being addressed by those who are not represented, who are not present in the ever-growing umbrella acronym for gender and sexual orientation rights to basic humanity. What we can acknowledge from the visibility of an acronym that has grown is that the commonality shared by different factions in the same movement is not enough to ensure the rights of those who experience the intersectionality of multiple oppressions until those truths are brought to the forefront. And when that happens the benefits achieved are palpable to all people in that specific movement. This holds true for the fat activist community as well. It is imperative that the voices of folks whose intersectionality of interwoven identities includes being a person of size are incorporated into the leadership of our shared commonality or sizeism will continue to flourish.

As we began to dialogue about the topic of being a WOC in a fat activist community, we realized that despite our quite different backgrounds we share a very common WOC experience of having the body hatred we experience from our cultural communities dismissed by a number of fat white activists. This is a repeated action we both keep running into—being told that we're lucky to come from cultures that embrace large women. First our background. Irene identifies as a fat black southern woman, and Juana emigrated from Mexico halfway through her childhood, becoming a U.S. citizen at the age of 18. We both realize that our experiences have formulated our knowledge; that no amount of research will make an academic have a deeper understanding of our realities than the validity of living it on a daily basis.

THE INVISIBLE WOMAN (OF COLOR)

Juana:

"Ay, ella me cae gorda." My body unconsciously tensed during the conversation as my average-sized feminist Mexican compatriot expressed that she couldn't stand a fellow coworker. When I expressed my distaste for the expression "She falls fat on me" as an indicator of dislike, I was met with the dismissive justification, "Oh, it's just a harmless saying." Harmless? In self-protection my fat body cringed as I resisted internalizing fat equals bad. Can a concept ingrained so deeply into the fabric of a society that it results in a common expression truly be free from repercussions to individuals manifesting that description?

During this same week a white fat activist told me I was lucky to be born into a culture that desired fat women, because she was tired of dealing with oppressive body size attitudes. Really? Because growing up in a culture that idealizes a woman's body as a size 8–10 rather than a size 4–6 is going to result in a significantly different experience for my then size 24 thighs? Is the inherent sexism in a woman's worth being equated to her body size any less oppressive simply because the number on the scale of acceptability is 20 pounds more?

In both scenarios I left the conversations feeling my experiences were not acknowledged. That someone who hadn't walked in my shoes was inaccurately interpreting the path that I walked, rendering my reality invisible. And in both cases a layer of self-protection developed. The loss of my emotional safety resulted in a loss for them as well. Because rather than collaborating to address our common areas of systemic oppression and to support each other in the areas that differed, I kept a sort of hypervigilant walking on eggshells around each of them so as not to be emotionally slapped in the face in that manner again.

Like all individuals, my identity and experiences is based on several factors. I cannot choose which of those to belong to, and while I have the ability to determine how I'll respond, I cannot choose to avoid being treated by others based on how they see me. Irene:

We were driving back from a concert when the conversation took "that turn." It is almost inevitable that it would happen. Get a room full of women together and it always seems to come to that topic. More negative in expression than positive in most cases but omnipresent. I think it comes from a lifetime of being told how to think about ourselves. A childhood where pretty slender princesses always got their prince, castle by the sea, and dainty if not dangerous glass high-heeled haute couture. The comparative discussion about weight where everyone weighs in with a heavy degree of shared self-shaming.

I think I was about 315 pounds at the time. The next heaviest person in the car was still able to shop comfortably at Abercrombie & Fitch. They were comparing their weight and dress sizes, talking about how gross they were. Each taking a turn saying how awful they looked and convincing each other that they were perfectly acceptable in size. It took a little bit but I finally got up the courage to say something.

"I am going to have to ask you to stop calling yourselves fat unless you actually are. I'm actually fat so to listen to you trash your bodies is really messed up."

There was a moment of silence followed by nervous laughter and half-hearted apologies. One of the travelers mistook my nice please shut up for staking the ultimate fat claim and in her misguided attempt to assuage me said, "It's okay for you though. Everyone likes fat black women."

I was stunned, speechless; my mind drew several blanks as it tried to stop reeling. Being the sole woman of color on that car ride and the only fatty, I was outnumbered. But even if I was not outnumbered, I was so confused by the exchange that I had absolutely no idea how to feel. All I was certain of was that something was wrong, rotten in the State of Denmark, wrong. I eventually stopped hanging out with those people and started hanging around with other fatties.

I felt safe. I felt like I could finally breathe and be okay with my body around other fat women.

I was mistaken

Another car ride

Another body-shaming party

Another plea to stop met with the assumption that because I'm black being fat affects me less.

It was infuriating.

This concept that my experience in this body is not as valid as another person's experience in a fat body. I was told that black men love fat women, and that fat black *women are all sassy creatures with great attitudes. After all Torrid had a T-shirt that said, "Everyone love a Black Chick," and it came in up to 4x so it had to be true. My sass and my attitude is not a superpower I gained when I reached 250-plus pounds. It is a defense mechanism constructed from being born invisible to a world that judges me upon the color of my skin and the size of my ass. My confidence is crucible forged. I still face the same struggles as white fatties, and my black prince has yet to show up and roll me off my feet. It came across like a heavy-handed slap to the face . . . the realization that even within the fat community I was still invisible.*

There is a mythos surrounding fat WOC.

While it is true that fat WOC are represented in the media as favored characters, it does not change the fact that we are mammies, housekeepers, best friends, comic relief, and side dishes.

The myth that black and Latino men desire fat women keeps being shoved in our faces as a sort of fat white woman oppression Olympics designed to insinuate we fat WOC have it so much easier.

It's a myth that is problematic for many reasons: the sexism/heterosexism in that the value of women lies in how physically attractive they are assessed to be, the hegemonic beliefs of invalidating the actual experiences of another by patronizingly informing them of what they're going through, and most of all it's problematic because it simply isn't true.

This microaggressive way of thinking diminishes fat WOC life experiences as human beings who have experienced fat shaming and silences their voices as activists. It creates an unspoken hierarchy of validation.

Breaking this myth allows us to become visible heard and seen as Women. It is a revelation to many that WOC undergo similar dehumanization. This is only one part of a multilevel. As we walk through life, we are impacted not only by women but by our skin color, our eye color, our hair and facial structures. It is a complex jigsaw fitted together. Each piece affecting the other but having its own powerful repercussions.

I wasn't called fat by the taxi driver that almost hit me. I was called a fat nigger.

INTERSECTIONALITY, WOMEN, AND COLOR

The concept of intersectionality explains that oppressions that may typically be seen as independent—for example, racism, homophobia, classicism, and sexism—actually interact to create multiple systems of oppression at the intersections of the marginalizations and the prejudices that keep them in place. For example, if a culture hires less, pays less, and promotes less due to race, size, and gender, then the lack of income that follows can lead all three groups to be the victim of classicism. If someone is a member of more than one of those groups, then the intersection of the oppressions can lead to even greater negative consequences.

Juana:

If passed over for a promotion, for example, it's difficult for me to figure out if it's because I'm fat or female or because I emigrated to the United States. And at the heart of it, does understanding the specific oppression at work in that instance change the outcome? At the end of the day I was passed over. My fat white friend has perhaps been passed over for a promotion because of her size and my feminist Mexican friend because of her ethnic background. But the result in both of those cases is the same: employment opportunities denied them because they aren't being given out based on merit. So rather than divide myself from them, it would behoove each of us to incorporate our histories that end up with the same resulting outcome to dismantle the oppressive glass ceilings. If only merits were considered, then we all win. As long as factors other than merits are in place, we are all held back because it allows for the acceptance of prejudice to be a determining factor in who gets what.

Irene:

Every time before I go in for an interview, I am filled with trepidation and dread. I wear my tightest spanx and my vertical pinstripe suit with the slimming pencil skirt. My look is meticulous, professional, sleek, modern, and "accessible." Not only do I feel the need to look smaller during these interviews, but I downplay my blackness. My natural kinky hair is hidden under a brownish-black wig with slick straight hair that has a slight undercurl, my large lips darkened. I do this because I really need this job, and if past experience has taught me anything, the smaller I look and the more adherent to a European beauty standard the more likely I am to be hired.

While I am often hired for a position and given excellent reviews, my true hurdle is promotions. Over the years I convinced myself that I was being paranoid. That if I did my work the best that I could and kept getting great reviews that I would be promoted. I was so sure that people could see past my fatness and recognize what great work I was doing. After all, two other fatties I knew at this same location got promotions; I just had to bide my time. I didn't start to become disillusioned until a woman under me got promoted above me. I had been there longer with more accomplishments. It was then that I noticed that all the other women who were promoted were white.

Through intersectionality, WOC bring a complex tool kit for dealing with discrimination. Any movement that doesn't have representation from everyone impacted by that marginalization may win a battle or two but fails to win the cause. If we want to eradicate sexism but only white women receive the benefit and WOC are still subjected to sexism, then women as a whole are impacted by that sexism. If we strive for rights—for example men of color have the right to vote but WOC can't vote—then people of color as a group are still held back.

As WOC, fat discrimination is not just fat discrimination.

To treat it as such is striking only two notes on what should be a chorused chord.

I am a woman

I am a fatty

I am a person of color

All of these intersectionalities weave throughout each other with such a powerful adherence that one cannot be separated from the other. Our interactions with the world are altered by all of these things.

FORCED ASSIMILATION

Society is constantly forcing fatties through a rhetoric of shame to conform to its beauty standards. Our collective cry rails against this injustice. We want the uniqueness of our bodies to be celebrated to respect. Whether our curves are large or small, we want to be treated with the same thoughtfulness given to any person. This is our battle cry to the world; then it should be nailed to the wall of our own home.

Irene:

It took my hair out the first time . . . clumps of it.

It burned like hot ice. I imagined my head a stack of smoke. How long was it? Fifteen or 20 minutes with that awful white girlish pink tinged stuff dripping to my ears and eating the flesh away. I remember it even now. God, the liberation I felt when she put my head "under the sink" to wash out that awful lye-based acid. It felt like relieving yourself after waiting a long long time. Crude, I know, but that is the truth. Such intense pleasure after all that pain. Every muscle in my body ached with release. It was like I was being worked over by a grand masseur. Well, that was until she started scrubbing my scalp to make sure it was all out. Her freshly French-tipped manicured nails ripped at the newly opened wounds at war against my untamable hair. I remember the salt tears running from my eyes as I tried desperately not to cry aloud. Over the years it got easier, more accustomed to the pain. Just one of my many penances for being black and a woman.

I would leave that parlor hours later and relish in the feeling of the wind running its finger through my sore scalp. I didn't mind the fact that I would not be able to play bare-headed in the rain, sweat, or worst of all go swimming. I was happy I was no longer nappy. I would swing my head back and forth until I saw stars swimming in the clouds. I would turn in mad circles just to see my hair move freely like all those shampoo commercials. Just as loose and easy as those blond skinny models. For five minutes I was in heaven on earth. Just five minutes because my mother yelled at me to get back in the car/house lest the strong southern humidity cause it to go back, all the way back . . . to Africa. And that would be a waste of her 30 dollars. For a week I would suffer sleeping on hard curlers, thinking to myself that if Jesus could stand a crown of thorns, I would at least stand this. By the second week the chemical burns would heal up. Mama would scratch my head and the scabs would float to the top of the black river and fall like snow onto my back and the dark blue towel across her lap.

By the end of the second week, I was fine, perfect at peace. My scalp had healed over and my hair still moved when the wind touched it. But by the fourth week, it no longer hung down and the thin comb would not pass through it. And my scalp began to itch unmercifully. My mother interrogated me about what I had been doing to my hair. The hairdresser laughed and said my hair will one day be able to "hold the perm" for up to six weeks once I was older (it never did). Unruly once more like an unbroken wild animal thing back in Africa, all the way back in Africa.

And so the process began again.

So I could look

just like

jane

As Women of Size we have intimate knowledge of how damaging forced assimilation can be. Some of us have at one point in our lives done dangerous things to conform to the size standard. Ostracization, mistreatment, and shaming have led us down some less than desirous paths in an attempt to be seen, heard, and respected as human beings. Without WOC leadership, WOC are placed in a position of forced assimilation. The impact that our cultural backgrounds has on our life experience is not considered and this devalues a person as a whole.

LEADERSHIP

Why is it important to include WOC in leadership in the fat activist movement?

Why is it important to include fat people in the fat activist movement?

When the White House brought together a task force to discuss people of size, the voices of people of size were lacking from the task force. Instead the task force was comprised of experts who have drunk the Kool-Aid, believed the current social mores, and the end result is a pathologization of fat people labeling all fat people as unhealthy who suffer from a medical diagnosis of obesity (which is now being labeled a disease regardless of how healthy the individual fat person is).

The White House Obesity Task Force focus is to eliminate childhood obesity in one generation. The genocide of an entire categorized group of people in a single generation is a terrifying goal. Would that same goal have been chosen if fat people's voices and actual unbiased research were included on that task force? What happens when the experiences of fat people are dismissed by controlling dominant culture?

Children of wonderful parents are taken away because the parents or the children possess a certain body mass index number; health care services are ineffective, inadequate, or unattainable; employment is impacted, making it more difficult to get a job and getting paid less when a job is obtained; and on a daily basis fat people are subjected to bullying going down the street, in the public places they work, the schools they attend, the television and other social media outlets that support this, as well as on the Web. Not to mention the stigma faced in the relationship and dating world. There are many sources that demonstrate all of this—yet the White House still has a goal of eliminating fat people. It's pretty clear that there is a need for fat activism to include fat voices—that no matter how supportive allied voices are, it's not enough.

There is no difference within the fat movement.

How is a fat white activist to determine what is in the best interest of fat WOC and the end result not be racist and patronizing? Will a fat white activist ensure there is literature written in Spanish or Japanese? Will a fat white activist comprehend the cultural nuances of a culture that isn't their own? Will they deny the differences, perhaps not even seeing them, rendering that fat WOC invisible? Or will they see the experiences and address them without considering the perspectives of how fat WOC want it responded to—and in the process marginalize fat WOC? Or will the fat white activist movement realize there needs to be space at the social justice leadership table for fat WOC to be seen and heard and determine how to address the intersectional marginalizations of our experiences?

A fat activist movement that doesn't incorporate WOC in leadership roles is unable to understand and therefore unable to address the experiences of fat WOC. Oh sure, there can be much debate and intellectual analysis, and similar to anthropologists who observe other cultures and interpret them through their own biased perspectives, they'll fail at the actual action of understanding what is really going on and the actual acting on solutions rather than discussions. The voices specifically of WOC (and while this chapter focuses specifically on WOC, we'd like to note that it's important to include the voices of fat men of color and fat nonbinary gender folks of color as well) are key to this conversation. WOC leaders are essential in making that voice heard.

Many people think of leadership as the ability to get others to help complete a task together. We would like to take it a step further. A leader is not just a point person who rallies others get the job done or blazes a trail into the vast unknown. A leader is also a healer. A person capable of ending conflict, soothing pain, and creating solutions out of an intimate knowledge of what it means to come from a place of marginalization, oppression, invisibility, forced assimilation, and diverse intersectionality. That is fundamental to the social influence mentioned above.

In a world where fatties are mistreated, our movement is our "home." It is our safe space. It is a place where we are inspired, empowered, and vulnerable. If the movement is our home, then the leaders are the "gatekeepers."

A WOC leader would understand that regardless of stereotypes, our experiences are altruistic. Having visible WOC leaders creates a safe space for a balanced meeting ground for all women within the movement. We do not feel safe in a space where we are not represented, where our unique story has not been told. We do not feel safe in a space where we do not see an empowered reflection of ourselves.

We must not let racism (unintentional or otherwise) derail fat activism. Fat acceptance is for everybody. We can only voice our own individual experiences and we do not presume to speak for all fat WOC. However, based on those interactions that we've personally been subjected to, we believe that fat humans of color are frequently alienated in white-dominated fat spaces, because such spaces frequently do not hold themselves accountable when engaging in actions or communication that result in cultural appropriation. There is a dearth of apologies and holding itself accountable. All too rarely is there an attempt to rectify the damage done by only centering the voices and experiences of white fat folks, while dismissing or not acknowledging those of fat folks of color. The result is that fat people of color become alienated from white fat acceptance movements. It is imperative to incorporate the experiences of fat WOC into fat acceptance movements that have traditionally excluded us by focusing only on white fat women, because until our needs and experiences are incorporated into the size positivity movements, the oppression of people based on body size remains. We're fat too and we're impacted by the marginalizations in similar and different ways than fat women who do not experience the intersection of racism. Without the integration of all fat people's experiences, there is no safer space.

So, why are WOC leaders needed in the fat activist movement?

The question itself is a an example of *why we need WOC in fat activism leadership roles*. People in privileged positions tend to want to maintain that privilege. How can you, for example, resist a sexist society if only males are in leadership roles in the feminist movements? Heterosexual folks don't initiate bills for gay marriage; cisgender folks in leadership don't lead to transgender rights in prisons; thin people despite being subject to the same vitriol of fat hatred spewed out by this society are not discriminated against because of it. The true experts of any movement are the individuals who are being marginalized by social mores. Anthropologists cannot remove their own preconceived biases in interpreting the civilizations they study, and a host of subconscious perspectives influence how we process and interpret information.

When the White House chose to discuss gay policies, they invited gay folks to the table. When they chose to discuss fat people, they invited only slender folks to the table to patronistically determine what is in our best interest. We are not children incompetent to figuring out what our needs are.

When WOC are left out of leadership positions, a movement fails to meet the needs of those left out. While this segment focuses specifically on WOC in the fat activist movement, it's important to note that this rule applies to other intersectioned segments. A fat activist movement without gay fat activists will fail to understand the way fat oppression impacts queer community, will fail to address it properly, and in the end will fail to liberate all fatties and there will still be fat marginalizations. Oppressions do not exist in a vacuum—they are not placed neatly side by side—they are intertwined and you can't unravel one oppression and leave another one to fester and hope the solution is achieved.

NOTE

1. Infoplease "The Wage Gap," accessed February 26, 2014, http://www.infoplease.com/ipa/A0763170.html.

15

The Pragmatic Attitude in Fat Activism: Race and Rhetoric in the Fat Acceptance Movement

Erec Smith

Modern racism, unlike past manifestations, seems more difficult to grasp, more insidious. It comes in the form of unconscious acts of privilege and "microaggressions"[1] that, drop by drop, can eventually fill one with mental and emotional trauma. The fat acceptance movement is not immune to such issues. When I hear people of color express frustration at inherent white prevalence in the movement, I am reminded of my own racism-induced frustrations and traumas induced by racist acts—both intentional and unintentional. However, we must not forget that the dynamics within the movement are not unrelated to the dynamics outside the movement: the racist and "sizest" hegemony fat activists work to revise. As a movement, we must work to remedy our internal issues without forgetting our real battle against external issues. I think the ability to do both may depend on a strong pragmatic attitude, one that acknowledges the confines of a particular situation while simultaneously working to break through them.

In 2012 NOLOSE,[2] a fat activism organization, published an open letter from the fat acceptance movement's people of color (POC) to its white members. The letter, "a response to white fat activism from People of Color in the fat justice movement," sees white privilege creating a rift within the movement, and demands that POC, who are being heavily targeted within antifat rhetoric, should have more of a voice. After charging the white fat activists with exclusivity within fat positive initiatives—specifically, the I Stand Against Weight Bullying initiative created as a response to Georgia's antifat and racist Stand4Life campaign—the movement's POC concluded the letter with a bulleted list of five demands:

- POC in the fat justice movement deserve thoughtful and clear discussions around not just the intention of diversity and inclusion in the work you wish to do, but also the actual impact of the work within communities of color.
- POC in the fat justice movement demand and deserve that white fat activists build authentic collaborations with communities of color and work as allies.
- POC in the fat justice movement demand and deserve allies showing up to the table of our campaigns and work, rather than constantly being told they have made a place for us at theirs.
- POC in the fat justice movement clarify that our allies will practice doing the work of learning about the histories and impacts of colonization and oppression on POC, seek other allies to learn from and with, be open to dialogue, taking feedback, and allowing people's firsthand experiences of racism to be the final and authoritative voice on the subject of impact to communities of color.
- POC in the fat justice movement offer that through the work of authentic inclusivity, singular vision will become shared vision. Coalition will happen. Bridges will be mended and built.[3]

I can stand behind most of these demands; however, I cannot say the same about the fourth bullet point, entirely. I strongly promote the self-education regarding oppression and an openness to honest dialogue, but the final request, to allow "people's firsthand experiences of racism to be the *final and authoritative* voice on the subject of impact to communities of color," seems tricky. My issue with this statement is not the dictatorial connotations of the term "final and authoritative" but the ideological eclecticism possible in "people's firsthand experiences." Based on my standpoint (which, like everyone's, is quite intersectional) and my firsthand experience with racism, I can understand the problem with white privilege inside the fat acceptance movement. However, that same experience leaves me conflicted about such things *outside* the movement, specifically the visual and communicative aspects of fat activism. My conflict may be presented best in the interrogative: How do we reconcile racial inclusivity within the fat acceptance movement with our need to combat the apparently racist and aesthetically exclusive initiatives outside of the movement? Is the prevalence of white people as the collective "face" of fat activism a more rhetorically and politically powerful public image for all those affected by antifat bias, or is such predominance too detrimental to race relations within the fat acceptance movement? I speculate that, from a rhetorical standpoint, the current white prevalence is somewhat understandable, but, from a pragmatic standpoint, all members of the fat acceptance movement must actively assess and reshape fat activism to move beyond this prevalence. Rhetoric and pragmatism, or their confluence—what James Berlin calls "social-epistemic rhetoric"—may be the antidote to issues of race, privilege, and exclusivity in the fat acceptance movement.

I want to illustrate my arrival at this conclusion by discussing how my "firsthand experiences" have shaped my subject position within and without fat acceptance. Based on this subject position, I arrive at a rhetorical analysis of what I call the American aesthetic Discourse that explains why white prevalence *outside* of the movement may be temporarily imperative. This idea may anger many people, and it should. Indeed, it angers *me*. Thus I conclude this chapter by promoting a "pragmatic attitude" and social-epistemic rhetoric to enhance shared leadership by white and POC fat activists to both acknowledge the temporality of an apparent white prevalence and develop the means to move toward a more inclusive and eclectic (and, therefore, ideal) fat acceptance movement.

How my "firsthand experience of racism" and other factors shape my viewpoint:

Marilyn Wann, in her foreword to the *Fat Studies Reader*, suggests that we all realize our subject positions in relation to the fat acceptance movement. We should be self-reflexive and acknowledge how our experiences influence our thoughts regarding fat activism.[4] So, perhaps my initial step should be a quick explanation of how my identified subject position, a conglomerate of my experiences with racism as well as experiences with my own privilege and personal interests, raises such conflicts for me. As I will explain, my intersectionality confirms that my "firsthand experience of racism" is connected to, and consubstantial with, other aspects of my subjectivity—aspects that are positions of privilege as well as nonprivilege.

To parse out aspects of my intersectionality I deem most relevant to the purpose of this chapter, I am a "not-fat," male, African American scholar of rhetoric.[5] By "not-fat," I denote my physical appearance because I am neither thin nor fat *by societal standards*. (That is, although my body mass index may be over 25, most people would not label me as fat upon looking at me. Also, I refrain from using terms like "average" because of the various interpretations of that word.) Based on being not-fat, I know I can support causes of fat liberation, write about my position within fat activism, and give my insights in attempts to inform people of the various perspectives regarding fat acceptance, but, ultimately, I must emphasize a need to *listen* and act accordingly to those who most embody this movement. As a not-fat *male*, I am double-privileged within a fat acceptance context. This movement consists mostly of women and always has. Fat men do suffer from weight discrimination but not nearly as much as women, who mainstream society wants to see as bastions of purity and virtue, features often associated with thinness.[6] As a not-fat male *of African American descent*, I can relate significantly to the irritation and frustration of dealing with those who do not realize their racial privilege. Also, I can discern the different "meanings" of body types, from an aesthetic viewpoint, found in African American communities. Lastly, as a not-fat, male, African American *rhetorician*, I am interested in the tropes used within discourse communities to either support or deride certain modes of thought or action. All these aspects intersect to create a subject position that engages in active listening, understands his own privilege, acknowledges his own experiences with racism, and embraces rhetoric analysis. Accordingly, I find the visual/rhetorical prevalence of white culture in fat activism as simultaneously unfortunate and strategic from a rhetorical and pragmatic perspective. Deeming such prevalence as unfortunate may be clear enough. However, its pragmatic and rhetorical efficacy may require more elaboration.

THE PRAGMATIC ATTITUDE

As a scholar of rhetoric, I am always cognizant of rhetorical context. Aristotle's definition of rhetoric, "an ability, in each [particular] case, to see the available means of persuasion,"[7] applies just as much to the fat acceptance movement as any other situation. Thus if one is to champion the acceptance of fat people in America, one would do well to frame fat people in an American context and act accordingly. While probing the "fat-o-sphere," reading relevant essays, and partaking in conversations about size acceptance, I see a predominance of white women from a wide socioeconomic range—and, based on current aspects of fat bias, that predominance can be construed as strategic. From the real-life players in the movement to the movement's graphic depictions meant to reflect pride and strength, the image of the fat, white female[8] may warrant more face time—*at this point*. Although the fat acceptance movement is meant to be inclusive and inviting, the rhetorical situation—one steeped in racial and socioeconomic stereotypes that fuel discrimination—may put most of the onus on white women to be the loudest and most visible members of the fat acceptance community.

The American tradition of pragmatism and its marriage to rhetoric inform my admittedly controversial assessment. Pragmatism, an attempt to "interpret each notion by tracing its respective practical consequences," shunning abstraction and insufficiency for "concreteness and adequacy,"[9] is an initiative for which constant dialogue unencumbered by the quest for a final solution is imperative. Like "rhetoric," the term "pragmatism" has many descriptions. However, for our purposes, Cornel West's description is most fitting:

> American Pragmatism is a diverse and heterogenous tradition. But its common denominator consists of a future-oriented instrumentalism that tries to deploy thought as a weapon to enable more effective action. Its basic

impulse is a plebian radicalism that fuels an antipatrician rebelliousness for the moral aim of enriching individuals and expanding democracy.[10]

West quickly admits that this tradition has had past issues with provincialism and ethnic exclusivity but arrives at a true and more inclusive definition of pragmatism that "is less a philosophical tradition putting forward solutions to perennial problems . . . and more a continuous cultural commentary or set of interpretations that attempt to explain America to itself *at a particular moment in time*"[11] (my emphasis).

Thus my position here is not to merely point out the obvious or to blame, complain, or let anyone off the hook, but to explain an approach dictated by our contemporary situation. I believe most fat activists are beyond discursive alienation and I believe the goals of whites and POC are similar enough to enable collaboration. So, in this chapter I want to suggest that we focus on "concreteness and adequacy" that can only ever be temporary, and this focus must manifest through dialogue in the spirit of what James Berlin calls social-epistemic rhetoric, a rhetoric that comes out of pragmatism and denotes "the study and critique of signifying practices in their relation to subject formation within the framework of economic, social, and political conditions"[12] I am not saying that white women should usurp leadership and organization within the movement. I am definitely not saying that white women are inherently superior to others in the movement. I do, however, think it imperative to accurately gauge the contemporary rhetorical context and act/dialogue accordingly. Based on my previously parsed subject position in the framework of what I call an American aesthetic Discourse, my analysis has drawn me to the pragmatic attitude: an approach to texts of any kind that shuns the search for a final or foundational methodology in exchange for methodologies contingent upon a given situation in time. According to Elizabeth Walker Mechling and Jay Mechling in "American Cultural Criticism in the Pragmatic Attitude," the pragmatic attitude involves, among other things, an assumption of the social construction of reality, a privileging of everyday experience and local knowledge, and a real desire to make a difference in the world.[13] Thus the pragmatic attitude brings me to the idea that the visual and rhetorical presence of the fat, white female in the fat acceptance movement may be a generally strategic move—even if unintentionally so—and an adherence to social-epistemic rhetoric can help those within the movement construct goals of inclusivity (and other goals) and strategies to achieve them.

THE AMERICAN AESTHETIC DISCOURSE

My deductions regarding the role of white women in fat activism may be better explained through considering the current aesthetic Discourse of

America. When using "Discourse," I abide by James Gee's definition of his intentionally capitalized term: a recognizable "identity kit" that integrates "words, acts, values, beliefs, attitudes, social identities, as well as gestures, glances, body positions and clothes."[14] The Discourse of American aesthetics often excludes non-Eurocentric ideals and typically excludes fat people. Abercrombie and Fitch CEO Mike Jeffries expressed this in no uncertain terms when questioned about the lack of "plus" sizes in his stores: "We go after the attractive all-American kid with a great attitude and a lot of friends," Jeffries said. "A lot of people don't belong [in our clothes], and they can't belong. Are we exclusionary? Absolutely."[15] Jeffries describes the dynamics of Gee's Discourse almost perfectly. Fat people "don't belong" and "can't belong" in the American aesthetic Discourse. Is this Discourse community, this "club" as theorists like Gee and Gerald Graff have called it, exclusionary? Yes, as exclusionary as Abercrombie and Fitch.

So, how does one begin to break into/break apart such an exclusionary club? Anthony Giddens, in *The Constitution of Society*, identifies three "structural dimensions of social systems": (1) Signification (symbolic action; language); (2) Legitimation (normative action); and (3) Domination (allocation or authorization of resources).[16] Although each dimension is significant to fat studies and fat activism,[17] I think the first step toward breaking down and revising exclusionary Discourse, and the initial explanation for my conclusion about white women's roles in fat acceptance, is that of Signification.

By Signification, Giddens denotes the way people interact with society through communicative practices: language, signs, images, etc.; these are all aspects of Gee's concept of Discourse. Each "identity kit" has distinct communicative practices—although they may overlap with other practices in other Discourses—that popularize, perpetuate, and strengthen the values of a particular Discourse community. According to this concept of Signification, within each Discourse certain signs and symbols are expected and others aren't. Mike Jeffries's "attractive, all-American" kid club does not expect a large minority presence and absolutely no fat presence. In fact, the symbols that aren't expected are either dismissed outright or "transmuted"—made sense of—as something quirky, odd, situational, etc. So, in the American aesthetic Discourse community—the network of the beautiful, typically white, middle-class, and definitely thin—fat is deemed undesirable.

What's more, within that same Discourse, the aesthetic sensibilities of marginalized people are deemed inferior—if not depraved. Images of proud fat women of a marginalized race would be "transmuted" into another example of that particular standpoint's utter difference and inferiority compared to the "normal" sensibilities of the American aesthetic Discourse. Amy Farrell, author of *Fat Shame*, provides an interesting explanation for this:

One of the key bodily signs of inferiority for scientists and thinkers of the 19th and early 20th centuries was fatness. . . . Fat became clearly identified as a physical trait that marked its bearers as people lower on the evolutionary and racial scale—African, "native" peoples, immigrants, criminals, and prostitutes. . . . Thin, in contrast, became identified as a physical trait of those higher on the evolutionary and racial scale—aristocrats, white people, men. Fatness, then, served as yet another attribute demarcating the divide between civilization and primitive cultures, whiteness and blackness, good and bad.[18] So, a proud, happy fat woman of African-American descent would be dismissed, or transmuted, as yet another example of how odd and uncivilized non-hegemonic cultures can be.

What's more, minority communities are at least *perceived* to be more comfortable with fat. Lonnae O'Neal Parker's article in the *Washington Post* reads, "although black women are heavier than their white counterparts, they report having appreciably higher levels of self-esteem"[19] (O'Neal Parker). It seems like their minority status protects them, in a way; hegemonic pressures don't affect them as much as they affect whites. The article continues, "The notion that all women must be culled into a single little-bitty aesthetic is just one more tyranny, they say. And black women have tools for resisting tyranny, especially from a mainstream culture that has historically presented them negatively, or not at all."

For reasons spanning from African roots to the freedom of marginalized societies to set their own standards, African Americans seem to traditionally have a different standard of beauty and femininity—one more accepting of plus sizes.[20] This standard—this alternative Discourse of aesthetics—did not go unnoticed by hegemonic powers. In fact, it is often used to further denigrate African Americans. For many white Americans, being thin is proof that one deserves to be white. As Farrell writes, thinness has been usurped by white culture as a way to separate themselves from cultures that do not put such an emphasis on fat or, completely adversely, praise fat bodies. However, a proud, happy, fat *white* woman exemplifying *every other* marker of the American aesthetic Discourse, i.e., Gee's "ways of using language, of thinking, feeling, believing, valuing, and of acting,"[21] is much harder to explain away.

The issue of race in fat studies and fat acceptance is quite salient. To white America, from the turn of the twentieth century to now, fat is deemed a characteristic of those less civilized or those whose cultures do not see fat as odd but as normal or at least acceptable, e.g., minority cultures.[22] What's more, in order to paint a negative picture of an opposing political group, one needs only to represent that group as fat and all its concomitant stereotypes: lazy, devious, undisciplined, etc.[23] For this reason, race is a heavily rhetorical aspect of the fat acceptance movement.

This issue is made even more poignant when considering the trend that athletic black women are often deemed unnatural and fat within the American Discourse of aesthetics. In the health-based web magazine *Frugivore*, Tamara Winfrey Harris's article, "Black, Female Athletes Still Too Big for the Mainstream," observes the derogatory opinions of accomplished and physically fit black athletes' bodies. She looks at the opinions about Serena Williams's physique and writes that the hegemonic verdict regarding black women's bodies "is not about our health and welfare, but exotification and the long-held belief that we are anti-women who lack the delicacy and femininity of other members of our gender."[24] It seems like black women, in general, already have too much going against them within aesthetic American Discourse.

But, what about white women? Although fat stigma is used against both minorities and whites, fat white people have a less obstructed path, since the human respect due to those minorities had already been systematically stripped from them. From a hegemonic standpoint, the place of fat stigma in minority communities can be understood as a subcategory of general racism: those minorities are "supposed" to be less than the mainstream culture; size is just one more reason to look down on them. To project fat stigma onto a white person, however, is to deem that person a letdown, a shame to the race, a pariah, a minority in hegemonic clothing. There is a correlation between thin and white in this country.[25] To be fat and white, though, is anomalous at best; at worst, it is a sign of failure as a white person.

Nevertheless, from a rhetorical standpoint, mainstream perceptions of fat body pride in minority communities may necessitate the fat, white female to be the "face" of size acceptance. If the mainstream already sees African Americans, for instance, as more inferior, any fat acceptance could be used as yet another sign of that inferiority. Their fat pride could be described as what British author Sara Bird calls "Fatorexia": a body "disorder" that denotes a fat person's denial that he or she is fat.[26] Paul Campos describes this phenomenon and its connotations in *The Obesity Myth: Why America's Obsession with Weight Is Hazardous to Your Health*, when he writes, "The single most noxious line of argument in the literature [of the obesity epidemic] is that black and Hispanic women need to be 'sensitized' to the 'fact' that they have inappropriately positive feelings about their bodies."[27] The image of white women exuding fat pride, however, may be much more agitating—and eye-opening— to those who would stigmatize fatness.

FAT ACCEPTANCE AND SOCIAL-EPISTEMIC RHETORIC

Again, my conclusions about the fat, white, female in fat activism are not to say that the movement is hers, alone. That would defeat the purpose. As a black person in America, I have suffered from various manifestations of racial discrimination. Despite a more improved racial climate, race relations are still less positive than they may often seem.[28] Thus I can significantly relate to the irritation and frustration of those in society who do not realize that they enjoy a bit of privilege. Peggy McIntosh, in "White Privilege and Male Privilege: A Personal Account of Coming to See Correspondences through Work in Women's Studies," writes that such ignorance "is kept strongly inculturated in the United States so as to maintain the myth of meritocracy, the myth that democratic choice is equally available to all." She goes on to write, "Keeping most people unaware that freedom of confident action is there for just a small number of people props up those in power, and serves to keep power in the hands of the same groups that have most of it already."[29] My conclusions about the role of fat white women in fat acceptance are not meant to perpetuate or justify white privilege. From a rhetorical standpoint, images of proud, white, fat women would probably do more to create a sea change in American aesthetic Discourse. The idea is that once the walls gating this Discourse community are jarred open, the rhetorical situation, and this perceived racial dynamic in the fat acceptance movement, may change.

I believe we can take a cue from scholarly perceptions and descriptions of third wave feminism. Shelly Budgeon, in *Third Wave Feminism and the Politics of Gender in Late Modernity*, writes that "third wave feminism advocates working with the particular differences that constitute women's positions at the local level, inviting the expression of hybrid identities, while developing strategies for working productively across differences based on a coalitional politics of affinity rather than equivalence."[30] At "the local level," which I read as a particular temporal situation (and, of course, a rhetorical situation), strategies may move in particular directions only to be reevaluated and re-moved when a new situation grows out of the current one. Maybe the current situation dictates that the white female is a salient symbol of fat acceptance, and maybe an appreciation of *kairos*, a specific rhetorical moment in time, will tell us when to alter that.

This, of course, is the pragmatic attitude, and the lingua franca of many who take on this attitude is social-epistemic rhetoric. According to James Berlin, social-epistemic rhetoric is one that acknowledges as communication "discovery and invention, not mere reproduction and transmission."[31] Most of all, social-epistemic rhetoric acknowledges the inherent ideologies reflected in all modes of communication and works with/around ideological disparities in discourse. Berlin writes,

> Social-epistemic rhetoric is self-reflexive, acknowledging its own rhetoricity, its own discursive constitution and limitations. This means that it does not deny its inescapable ideological predispositions, its politically situated condition. It does not claim to be above ideology,

a transcendent discourse that objectively adjudicates competing ideological claims. It knows that it is itself ideologically situated, itself an
intervention in the political process, as are all rhetorics. Significantly,
it contains within it a utopian moment, a conception of the good
democratic society and the good life for all its members. *At the same time,
it is aware of its historical contingency, of its limitations and incompleteness,
remaining open to change and revision.*[32] (my emphasis)

Ultimately, to take the pragmatic attitude and participate in social-epistemic
rhetoric, one must not be satisfied with any particular strategy beyond its
immediate use. To put it simply, what works today may not work tomorrow.
Or, what worked this morning may not work this afternoon. Constant
dialogue that acknowledges the myriad contingencies of circumstance and
subject position is the best way to figure that out.

Deciding what works and what doesn't has to be discussed with significant
frames in mind, like American aesthetic Discourse. Thus fat activists
must negotiate discourse within the movement to deal with the decidedly
oppressive American aesthetic Discourse. Echoing Giddens's concept of
Signification and motivated by Stuart Hall's take on the term, Berlin writes
that signification is "a material force that must be studied in its complex operations of enforcing and challenging power arrangements. Social-epistemic
rhetoric is in accord with this perspective ... persuasion in the play of power
is at the center of this rhetoric, and studying the operation of signifying practices within their economic and political frames is the work it undertakes."[33]

The work of social-epistemic rhetoric, within and among Discourses, is a
negotiation of subject position, as well. This was the problem with mere social
constructionist rhetoric, which often inadvertently silenced people unrecog-
nized by those enjoying identified subject positions. One must either take on
an "identified subject position," one that seems to fit comfortably in a particular Discourse,[34] or take on a "subversive subject position" that brings an identified subject position from another Discourse to oppose the forces denying
access to agency in the current Discourse.[35] Social-epistemic rhetoric
welcomes negotiations of subject positions and anticipates—hopes for—
subversive subject positions to present themselves in ways that enhance the
concreteness and adequacy of a particular moment.

To clarify, the rhetorical analysis of antifat bias inherent in the American
aesthetic Discourse may explain the current role of white women in fat activism, but the pragmatic attitude and social-epistemic rhetoric may help one see
its efficacy, its temporality, and the ways to revise it toward more inclusivity.
Let me make clear that fat activism must be an all-inclusive movement if it
is going to work, a movement dedicated to a process dependent on dialogue,
self-reflexivity, and trust in local, everyday knowledge. The demands of POC

in "a response to white fat activism from People of Color in the fat justice movement" definitely promote such necessities. In fact, this strategy will ideally move beyond race and ethnicity. In an online conversation thread in March, a fat and disabled person said in response to the NOLOSE.org letter that "my motto has always been Solidarity at Every Size . . . and my understanding is that solidarity is a process, not a destination. Letters like this add to my knowledge and understanding, and help move things forward in general."[36] If solidarity is a process and not a destination, perhaps every step we make to promote self-pride and fight discrimination, regardless of any group affiliation among fat activists, is a step toward fat acceptance in society AND solidarity within the movement.

NOTES

1. Microaggressions are everyday slights and insults performed by well-intentioned people. See Derald Wing Sue and David Rivera "Microaggressions in Everyday Life," *Psychology Today*, October 5, 2010, http://www.psychologytoday.com/blog/microaggressions-in-everyday-life/201010/racial-microaggressions-in-everyday-life.

2. "NOLOSE is a volunteer-run organization dedicated to ending the oppression of fat people and creating vibrant fat queer culture" (http://www.nolose.org/about/who.php).

3. Tara Shuai et al., "A response to white fat activism from People of Color in the fat justice movement," NOLOSE, 2012, http://www.nolose.org/activism/POC.php.

4. Marilyn Wann, "Foreword," in *The Fat Studies Reader*, ed. Esther Rothblum and Sondra Solovay (New York: New York University Press, 2009), ix.

5. I do not include socioeconomic status or sexual orientation for brevity's sake. Although both demographics are important, I believe I can elucidate sufficiently without them. Both statuses must be taken up at some point.

6. Peter Stearns, *Fat History: Bodies and Beauty in the Modern West* (New York: New York University Press, 1997), 77–78.

7. Aristotle, *On Rhetoric*, trans. George A. Kennedy (New York: Oxford University Press, 1991), 36.

8. Although both men and women suffer from fat shame, women of all ages seem to pay the bigger price. See Rebecca Pearl, Rebecca Puhl, and Kelly Brownell, "Positive Media Portrayals of Obese Persons: Impact on Attitudes and Image Preference," *Health Psychology* 31, no. 6 (2012): 821–29.

9. William James, *Pragmatism and Other Essays* (New York: Washington Square Press, 1963), 25.

10. Cornel West, *The American Evasion of Philosophy: A Genealogy of Pragmatism* (Madison: University of Wisconsin Press, 1989), 5.

11. Ibid.

12. James Berlin, *Rhetorics, Poetics, and Cultures* (Urbana, IL: NCTE, 1996), 77.

13. Elizabeth Walker Mechling and Jay Mechling, "American Cultural Criticism in the Pragmatic Attitude," in *At the Intersection: Cultural Studies and Rhetorical Studies*, ed. Thomas Rosteck (New York: Guilford Press, 1999), 140–50.

14. James Paul Gee, *Social Linguistics and Literacies: Ideologies in Discourse* (Bristol, PA: Falmer Press, 1990), 142.

15. Benoit Denizet-Lewis, "The Man Behind Abercrombie & Fitch," *Salon*, January 24, 2006, http://www.salon.com/2006/01/24/jeffries/.

16. Anthony Giddens, *The Constitution of Society* (Los Angeles: University of California Press, 1984).

17. I briefly discuss the relevance of "Legitimation" and "Domination" at http://www.moreofmetolove.com.

18. Amy Farrell, *Fat Shame: Stigma and the Fat Body in American Culture*, Kindle ed. (New York: New York University Press, 2011), chap. 3.

19. Lonnae O'Neal Parker, "Black Women Heavier and Happier with Their Bodies than White Women, Poll Finds," *Washington Post*, February 27, 2012, http://articles.washingtonpost.com/2012-02-27/lifestyle/35445428_1_black-women-white-women-african-american-women.

20. Stearns, *Fat History*, 92.

21. Gee, *Social Linguistics and Literacies*, 143.

22. Farrell, *Fat Shame*, Kindle ed., chap. 3.

23. Ibid.

24. Tamara Winfrey-Harris, "Black, Female Athletes Still Too Big for the Mainstream," *Frugivore*, July 10, 2012, http://frugivoremag.com/2012/07/black-female-athletes-still-too-big-for-the-mainstream/.

25. Paul Campos, *The Obesity Myth: Why America's Obsession with Weight Is Hazardous to Your Health* (New York: Gotham Books, 2004), 81.

26. "What Is Fatorexia," *The Fatorexia Foundation*, http://fatorexia.org/.

27. Campos, *The Obesity Myth*, 88.

28. Charles A. Gallagher, "Color-Blind Privilege: The Social and Political Functions of Erasing the Color Line," in *Rethinking the Color Line: Readings in Race and Ethnicity*, ed. Charles A. Gallagher, 2nd ed. Chapter 13, pages 130–142 (New York: McGraw-Hill, 2004).

29. Peggy McIntosh, "White Privilege and Male Privilege: A Personal Account of Coming to See Correspondences through Work in Women's Studies," in *Privilege: A Reader*, ed. Michael S. Kimmel and Abby L. Ferber (New York: Basic Books, 2003), 159.

30. Shelly Budgeon, *Third Wave Feminism and the Political of Gender in Late Modernity* (Hampshire, UK: Palgrave Macmillan, 2011), 5.

31. Berlin, *Rhetorics, Poetics, and Culture*, 81.

32. Ibid.

33. Ibid., 83.

34. Barry Brummett and Detine L. Bowers, "Subject Positions as a Site of Rhetorical Struggle: Representing African Americans," in *At the Intersection: Cultural Studies and Rhetorical Studies*, ed. Thomas Rosteck (New York: Guilford Press, 1999), 118.

35. Ibid., 119.

36. Sprinkles McGillicuddy, "Marilyn Wann: Here's Something Totally Fabulous and Crucially Needed!," Marilyn Wann, online posting to Facebook, March 13, 2012, https://www.facebook.com/marilynwann.

16

Black Women in Fat Activism

Rev. Dr. E-K Daufin

"Into Each Life Some Rain Must Fall" is the title of a 1944 top Harlem Hit Parade and pop chart song. Allan Roberts wrote it. The Ink Spots performed it as a duet, featuring Ella Fitzgerald and Billy Kenny.[1] "Into Each Life Some Rain Must Fall" is also a good way to say that the human condition provides for everyone some type of challenge to overcome. However, some groups who are not afforded much or any unearned privilege are likely to have many more challenges in addition to the whole range of human heartache.

The Black Women's Health Study of Boston University's Slone Epidemiological Center is the only long-term study of black women's health.[2] I am one of the closed group of 59,000 women who agreed in 1995 to participate in the study, which does a biannual follow-up on different topics. Though there are people of color on the advisory board, the principal investigators are three white women, Lynn Rosenberg and Julie Palmer from Boston University and Lucile Adams-Campbell from Georgetown University's Lombardi Comprehensive Cancer Center.[3]

National Public Radio reports that the Black Women's Health Study finds that genes, diet, socioeconomic status, and environmental factors conspire to make African American women the heaviest of United Statesians.[4] The report notes that experiencing white supremacy/racism correlates with African American women's higher weights, as do childbearing, having less access to safe affordable housing and exercise, quality affordable grocery stores, and lower rates of breast feeding than white women and Latinas.

The American Psychological Association and the Association of Black Psychologists reported that although higher educational status and more education seem "to somewhat protect" white women and Latinas from "rising obesity rates," education doesn't protect African American women.[5] They also agree that the "chronic stress of racism and caring for whole family systems" contributes to black women's obesity rates.

In fat activism we are concerned about ending unjustified, damaging weight stigma and discrimination, a part of which is educating the public about the multiple reasons for higher weights that have nothing to do with laziness, greed, or "lack of self-control."

For most black women—life "ain't been no crystal stair," to quote Langston Hughes's iconic Harlem Renaissance poem "Mother to Son."[6] In addition to the challenges most humans face as we all have to climb "the stairs of life," black women must contend with white supremacy, patriarchy/sexism, *and* size-ism at the institutional or structural *and* the personal levels. This chapter explores the intersectional challenges of African American women in fat activism. It also makes the case to African American and other women of color of all sizes to join the fat activism movement and take on leadership roles despite the many challenges. The chapter also outlines some ways in which white members of the movement can facilitate and support increasing the numbers of black and other women of color to enter the fat activism move-ment, take on leadership roles, and enhance their ability to persevere.

VOCABULARY

When I use the term "white supremacy," I'm not talking about the Ku Klux Klan here. Rather I refer to the pervasive notion that all things Caucasian are the norm, if not better than everything associated with other races—the stan-dard by which we all are judged. White supremacy is more inclusive than the word "racism" because it accounts for internalized, institutional, and personal racism. In addition, it accounts for the elements of "colorism," the discrimina-tion against those who have darker skin, darker hair color, kinkier hair tex-ture, slanted/so-called double-lidded eyes, and more "Africanized" facial features (wider noses with flat bridges, bigger lips, etc.). The white supremacist race hierarchy in the United States in general places all people of color below whites and all races above African Americans.[7]

Also, considering that African American women are the fattest population in the country[8] at over 82 percent of all black women, followed by Latinas at almost 76 percent,[9] weight discrimination also has an element of white supremacy. Higher weights among American Indian women varies widely according to the nation (preferred term over the word "tribe") from 26 to 81 percent according to a 1999 report.[10] The most recent 2010 Centers for Disease Control survey on higher and highest weights according to ethnicity does not have gender breakdowns but reports the rate for American Indians/ Alaskan Natives and Hawai'ians/Pacific Islanders at about 40 percent and Asians at 12 percent.[11] Though nearly 60 percent of white women are fat,[12] white women and Asian women are the thinnest women in the country.

For the record, when I use the word "patriarchy," I mean the notion that what is normal and good is that which is associated with men. It's a more accurate term than "sexism." *Heterosexism* is the notion that the only sexual orientation is heterosexual, and cisgender is part of patriarchy in that cisgender male/female pairings, traditionally where the male is dominant, are part of the normalized, or "wholesome," patriarchal system.

Fat discrimination/sizeism is inherently patriarchal because women naturally have a higher percentage of body fat to support childbearing and other hormonal functions.[13] Men must have 2 to 5 percent "essential" body fat, whereas women need to have 10 to 13 percent essential body fat.[14] Thus if the predominant culture considers fat to be evil, and it does, women are by necessity more "evil" than men.

Likewise, "sizeism" is the notion that everything good is associated with a slim body, including intelligence, sexiness, health, fitness, beauty, grace, attractiveness, self-control, and other positive attributes. I prefer the terms "higher and highest weight(s)" to those of "overweight" ("Over *what* weight?" I usually say when someone uses that term.), or "obese" (a loaded, medical diagnosis based on the way someone looks). The term "fat" I, as does the fat acceptance movement, use as a neutral or even positive reframing of what has been a pejorative description in the mainstream culture. Sizeism disproportionately negatively affects women of all colors compared to men, Latinas, and some American Indian women more profoundly and African American women the most.

"Negro" used to be the preferred term for African Americans while "black" was an insult. The Black Power movement helped the nation reclaim the term, as fat activism or fat liberation is holding up the fine, fierce adjective of "fat." Just as black can be a positive term, so may fat, used by the right person in the right way, be a positive term . . . or at least that's part of what we're working toward. The effect of using the term "fat" often changes according who says it and how, just as does the effect of using the word "black." Whenever possible I use the more inclusive term "Latina/Latino" to describe that ethnicity as a collective group, rather than by country (because those breakdowns are not widely available). "Hispanic" refers more accurately to natives of Spain living in the United States.[15]

I use the terms "African American" and "black" interchangeably. I am African American Indian identified. I am a quarter-blood Chiricahua Apache. However, those ancestors were urban Indians whose nation bonds were broken by colonialism and slavery. My American Indian ancestors often sought to disassociate themselves from the even more punitive African American identification. U.S. inhabitants are not the only "Americans," as all the land in the Western Hemisphere is "America" or the Americas. Most *United Statesian* people would visually identify me as a medium-to-light-brown-skinned African

American with fairly kinky hair and Anglo facial features. Those descriptors characterize my experience. Most of this chapter is therefore about African American women specifically.

My showing up often constitutes the only "racial integration" in otherwise all-white groups. In my life as a black woman in an "integrated" United Statesian world, I have to repeatedly correct the linear perception of those white people who ask me if I have "more trouble" with white supremacy *or* patriarchy. This problem even extends to some white faculty who teach at Historically Black Colleges and Universities (HBCUs) as I do. I can't separate my race from my gender. The two overlap and often compound the white supremacy and patriarchy with which I must contend.

Contrary to popular myth, you probably know by now that there is no effective, permanent weight loss diet or exercise regime for 95 percent of those of us who try them. In fact most of us who go from diet to diet seeking escape from weight stigma, harassment, and worse wind up *gaining* weight as our bodies recover from our bouts of starvation. Our brains add a little more padding to protect against the next weight loss diet, which our bodies read as the next "famine."[16]

So you know that the road to higher weights is complex and varied, but body mass index is 50 to 90 percent genetic.[17] Once one is at a higher weight, it's pretty much another unchangeable (within a narrow range of about 10–15 pounds)[18] demographic in the long term, similar to gender and race/ethnicity. I have been involved in the *fat acceptance movement* for most of my adult life. I define "fat activism" as different from fat acceptance perhaps in only degree. Activism insinuates *purposeful behavior* that seeks to enlarge the sphere of fat acceptance and decrease sizeism not only in one's self but also in the broader society.

FAT ACTIVISM IMPEDIMENTS FOR BLACK WOMEN

To review, 80 percent of African American women are at higher weights compared to 60 percent of white women. African American women make up about 7 percent of the United Statesian population.[19] African American women at higher weights are discriminated against on multiple levels. So why aren't black women at least 6 percent (roughly 80% of the 7% of the general population) of the fat acceptance movement and leadership? It may be for the same reasons that all fat white and other race women are *not* part of the fat acceptance movement and leadership.

It would be logical for at least all *fat* people to be part of the fat activism movement. But we're not. Too many of us don't know about the movement, or have too deeply internalized weight stigma before we discover there is such a thing as fat acceptance, much less activism.

Another reason more black women aren't a part of the fat acceptance movement may be related to the fact that "African-Americans are the most religiously devout racial group in the nation when it comes to attending services, praying and believing that [author's note: a thin or muscular, male, patriarchal] God exists,"[20] according to a 2007 Pew Research Center's Forum on Religion and Public Life report. This is coupled with the understanding that Christianity, particularly fundamental Christianity, is also often used to promote the ideas that (1) fatness is a sin resulting in failing to fight the Devil's temptation; (2) thinness is a gauge of one's relationship to Christ; (3) dieting is a way to salvation as a godly fight against evil, all equaling the misguided notion that thinness is next to godliness.[21]

A "healthy" diet or eating intuitively/mindfully and exercising regularly are good for you, will probably make you healthier, but won't make you much thinner and may even make you heavier, as most fat activism advocates know. It would benefit perhaps those of all colors and weights to be aware of and adopt the Health at Every Size perspective, which is an important part of the fat acceptance movement. Health at Every Size has five basic tenets: (1) enhancing health, (2) size and self-acceptance, (3) the pleasure of eating well, (4) the joy of movement, and (5) an end to weight bias.[22]

In addition, some reasons black women don't make up at least 6 percent of the fat acceptance movement may be the same as why black women, 100 percent of us *female*, don't make up 7 percent of the feminist movement. "Black women who participated in the Black Liberation Movement and the Women's Movement were often discriminated against sexually and racially. Although neither all the Black men, nor all the White women in their respective movements were sexist and racist, enough of those with powerful influence were able to make the lives of the Black women in these groups almost unbearable."[23]

Also, some myths acting as impediments to the participation of black women in the size acceptance movement and their taking leadership roles in fat activism are similar to the myths that diverted black women from joining the feminist movement.

These *myths* include:

1. The black fat woman faces no weight discrimination in the black community.
2. Racism is the primary or only oppression fat black women have to confront in the mainstream community.
3. The black fat woman faces no race discrimination in the size acceptance community.
4. Fat acceptance issues are narrow, apolitical concerns. Fat black women need to deal with the "larger struggle."

5. The fat acceptance movement's affiliation to other oppressed, stigma-tized, "fringed" communities discredits the movement.[24]

This chapter seeks to illuminate and defuse these myths. It is frustrating when size discrimination-sensitive, otherwise intelligent white people in the size acceptance movement ask me whether I have more difficulty as a black woman *or* as a fat woman. I have got to deal with the negative assumptions others make about me because of all three characteristics (female, black, *and* fat) at once. Virtually everyone in the fat acceptance movement knows that being fat is a fairly permanent state. However, many still don't understand that weight stigma is an *added* layer of pain, discrimination, and challenge for women of color, especially black women.

TRICKSTER AT THE CROSSROADS: THE BIG BLACK WOMAN BEAT DOWN

One of the world's greatest and most interesting trickster/chaotic figures is Eshu-Elegbara, one of the *Orisha*, the West African deities who are worshiped in many related forms across Africa and the African diaspora in the New World. While She/He embodies many obvious trickster elements—deceit for your own good, humor, sexuality, living outside the boundaries of human law—Eshu-Elegbara is also the god/goddess of communication and spiritual language. She/He is the gatekeeper between the realms of humans and gods, the tangled lines of force that make up the cosmic interface. Her/"His sign is the crossroads."[25]

We stand at Eshu's crossroads when we communicate about social justice issues that are intersectional and multilayered for those of us who are of more than one of the groups typically discriminated against, or of whom the main-stream culture holds prejudiced opinions and negative stereotypes. When I talk about privilege, I am referring to *unearned* privilege—the type of privi-lege you never asked for, or perhaps are even aware of, but you get because you show up in life as a member of a positively perceived, normative group.

For example, I was at a program in Northern California, working to help ease the crippling back pain that had almost taken me out of my livelihood and, as a woman with no support network, removed my ability to survive at all. All the men at the workshop were over 30 and married. The women were over 30, most single, and though beautiful, loveable, and talented in our own ways, none of us would be mistaken for a supermodel. One quarter-blood American Indian woman who looked 100 percent Irish and I, an African American who is also quarter-blood American Indian but looks distinctly African American, were the highest-weight people in the otherwise all-white group.

On the second day of the program, a new participant arrived. She was a 20-something, German-born, Nordic-looking blonde with blue eyes, a fashionably thin woman with big breasts. I was astounded by how invisible all the other women became to the men once this woman showed up.

For example, while seated at the long cafeteria table, I asked for someone to please pass the salt. I spoke clearly and loudly enough to be heard above the conversation, what little there was. No one seemed to hear me. Everyone just kept eating. I asked again and waited. Nothing. I got up, walked down the table to get the salt. A few moments later, the blond, white, thin, younger woman simply mentioned to no one in particular that her "eggs needed salt." Three men actually fell over themselves reaching for different salt shakers. One ran from about five places down the table. Another grabbed the salt shaker I had had to get for myself a few moments ago and handed it to her. It looked like a scene from a sitcom, but there was nothing funny about the feelings their behavior evoked in those of us straight women whom the men did not consider as attractive as the blond woman.

I don't think she even said thank you to all the swift salt servers. The next day at the same workshop, I dove into a freezing cold mountain pool of water. The men paid no attention, though I announced the decision and everyone obviously saw me do it. Fewer than five minutes later, the younger blond woman walked over and dove in. The men not only watched her every move but shouted words of encouragement and then praised her for her efforts. I asked them why they hadn't done the same for me a few minutes earlier. They were basically embarrassed and speechless. My objection didn't stop either the unearned privilege the men extended to her as the workshop progressed or her obvious familiarity with and expectation of that kind of positive support, attention, or response all the men gave to her.

Three of the white members said during a break that all aid to the poor should be cut because, "Those people don't want to work." One of the very nice white male counselors complained that his shoulder hurt after helping 11 other people together lift me in a trust exercise. So you see, virtually no experience is free of weight, race, and gender bias.

These were not cruel people. To the contrary, they were fairly aware and were at the workshop to become more sensitive and psychologically whole. Most of them seemed to like me. Still, all the women became faceless nonpersons when a woman with lots of unearned privilege showed up. She didn't ask others to treat her with great deference but didn't seem to notice that they always did. This was not in a fat activism community, but pretty much the same thing happens to higher-weight black women in many fat activism groups as we fight the unearned privilege the culture bestows so freely and ever increasingly upon those of lower weights. The white fat activism board members in the next example also were not cruel and would not have identified themselves as white supremacist or patriarchal.

Many years ago, I resigned from a national fat activism group as their African American community liaison because an African American male fat admirer stalked and harassed me at the conference. I called hotel security more than once about this member's harassment at the conference. When I got home, I made my case in writing to the association's then all-white, mixed-gender board of directors to censure this member in order to protect me at future conferences. Their published bylaws said his behavior was unacceptable and that anyone who behaved that way would be censured. Over the objections of the organization's white, female president, the board decided that the straight, African American male, fat-admirer member who flirted with the white women at socials was more valuable to the organization than me—a straight, female, African American fat woman who worked as a speaker, advocate, and consultant for them for free, even traveling at my own expense.

The director, with regret, told me the board said I could resign if I chose but they weren't going to write even a warning letter to the harasser, much less censure him. Though that board seemed to think that a fat black woman activism worker was worth a dime a dozen, I was one of only three African American women who I had seen in five years to even attend their national conferences, much less take on a leadership position.

I dropped out of fat activism leadership because I felt so devalued by the often unintentional, but nonetheless painful and isolating, white supremacy and patriarchy to which I was subject in what was then the largest fat activism organization I could find. Yet as recently as the year of this writing, I have experienced black men in fat activism forums treat white fat women those men had never met before with great positive attention and even gifts. Those same black men treated me and the few other black women at the conference as if we did not exist.

SOCIAL DISCRIMINATION AGAINST FAT BLACK WOMEN

Both the historical example and the more recent one of how white supremacy, patriarchy, and size all functioned as intersecting oppressions of black women are double-edged. Remember that these intersecting, multilayered, additional challenges also affect fat black women in health care, the workplace, school, and even church. Not only do the two social examples previously mentioned demonstrate how patriarchal influences contributed to the fat acceptance organization's board valuing a black male over a black female, both examples also touch on the delicate issue of our cultural glorification of white women as the very best and virtually only romantic partners for men of every race.

In the recent example, several fat white women at the conference to whom the black man had been so deferential were exclaiming to me how sweet and wonderful he was. Only when I brought to their attention that he had not treated me with the same attention and kindness did they quietly exclaim, "Ooooooh." They had not noticed, but as I pointed out examples, they agreed my observations were accurate.

In the older example, the black man was so valued by the fat activism organization because he flirted with the white women at the conference. Some fat activism publications even used to advise fat white women to seek out black and brown men for romantic partners. These publications and many white people in the fat activism movement misinterpret the great enthusiasm with which some black and Latino men may treat fat white women as a cultural, race-neutral supposed preference men of color have for all women of size. When the same black and Latino men do not respond as enthusiastically to black and Latina women of higher weights, those men are usually enacting white supremacy rather than a race-neutral attraction to fat women.

Contrary to popular white opinion, both within and outside of the size acceptance movement, black fat women face considerable social, political, economic, health care, and other discrimination in the black community as well as in the white or integrated world. This discrimination is in addition to the oppression we may encounter as females, African Americans or other races and ethnicities, class, skin, eye and hair textures, facial features, height, etc.

Unfortunately, the few grossly misguided black women who say black women *want* to be fat[26] as a means of purposeful defiance or other reasons of choice are the ones most publicized in mainstream media. Perhaps that is true of all progressive ideas. The person of the oppressed group who is willing to be a weapon of her own oppression is more readily accepted and promoted than those who would work to end the oppression that bears down upon them.

Perhaps all fat activism workers of every color have faced a thinner person who has no idea of the weight stigma fat people suffer. These naive thin people may claim that someone in her family or a potential romantic partner has said she was too thin and that equates with all the weight-based discrimination fat people face. Some African American women who are much smaller than the American mainstream average size 14–16 may hear remarks from an individual that they are too thin. However, as one fat black female responded to an article promoting the ignorant fat-black-women-are-fat-because-they-want-to-be rhetoric, "We know good and well they're not talking about having a little something extra in all the 'right' places, they're talking about [higher- and highest-weight women]."[27]

I agree with a black woman's lifestyle magazine's letter to the editor writer when she says, "Every time another study comes out about obesity in America or Black women's happiness being heavy, a slew of articles come out explaining why we're bigger than White women and why we're okay with that. It seems to me if we were really okay with it there'd be no need to explain anything."[28] I argue that studies that show black women are subject to no weight stigma, or are less psychologically affected by weight stigma than white women, are methodologically flawed.[29]

This popular myth that black fat women suffer no weight-based discrimination leads many black girls and women to be undiagnosed for many health concerns. (Fat activists know that higher weights in and of themselves are *not* health concerns.) Stephanie Covington Armstrong , author of one of the few books about an African American woman with bulimia, the autobiographical *Not All Black Girls Know How to Eat: A Story of Bulimia*, unfortunately stigmatizes fat bodies. She also takes a 12-Step/food addiction perspective rather than the more helpful, less stigmatizing Health at Every Size approach.[30] However, Dr. Deb Burgard, a white, Harvard-trained author, fat activist par excellence, and clinical psychologist says, as do many dieticians and social workers in the Association for Size Diversity and Health, that it's often difficult to get treatment for African American female bulimics and anorexics because we present with the disorders at higher weights than white females do.

Of course those who understand disordered eating know that weight loss dieting is also disordered eating. Fat white women have a hard time convincing health professionals and even family members that weight loss dieting is physiologically unsustainable and doesn't work in the long run or sometimes at all. There is a saying often attributed to Albert Einstein: "The definition of insanity is doing the same thing over and over again and expecting different results." Unfortunately, the weight loss industry and popular culture don't think that applies to dieting and weight loss efforts. Race stigma may make it even more difficult for fat black women to convince anyone that they exercise and "eat right."

Virtually all the crossover (popular with white audiences as well as black) African American mega-star sex symbols such as Beyoncé, Halle Berry, and Mariah Carey are smaller-than-average black women if not a supermodel/white actress size 0. Also every black woman top-of-the-chart recording artist and the throngs of black women in black-oriented music videos are relatively thin.[31]

"Even after the Black is Beautiful seventies, it is still the case that when African American woman are upheld as beautiful in the popular media, they usually have lighter skin, longer hair, and thinner body types that adhere more closely to those dominant standards"—the "narrowly defined beauty ideals based on Euro-American [white] aesthetics that are so firmly entrenched in this culture."[32] Black comedians denigrate higher-weight black women in both stand-up acts and feature films. Take any *Big Mama*, Tyler Perry/Madea movie or Eddie Murphy's *Norbit* as examples. I and most black fat women face weight-based prejudice from black and other race medical professionals, employers, students, teachers, coworkers, our families, potential suitors, etc.

Rare exceptions are hard-won and only partial victories. The Honey Beez are a seven-member, plus-size dance troupe that sometimes appears with the marching band (The Mighty Marching Hornets) at the Historically Black University where I am a professor of communication. The Honey Beez even had a national television appearance on the *Steve Harvey Show* last year.[33] Bands Director Dr. James Oliver founded the team after several plus-size black female students told him how they were survivors of weight-based bullying, from kindergarten through college. He says he decided to show people that in addition to being higher- and highest-weight young black women averaging 230 pounds, they also have "great athletic prowess, amazing routines, dexterity and joy for life."[34] Though many audience members laugh at the big-sized dancers at performances, by the time the Honey Beez do their signature running cartwheel to a split, most of the jeers turn to cheers.

The Honey Beez say that when they speak at local predominantly black high schools, the girls in the audience often contact them after the appearance to ask for advice on how to survive weight-based bullying.[35] Though the Honey Beez are one of a handful of plus-size dance teams at HBCUs, where black women outnumber black men 3 to 2,[36] and 8 out of 10 of the women are at higher weights, HBCUs are *not* a size-acceptance-positive community.

The Honey Beez and similar organizations were established by brave, loving individuals *because* of the need to combat weight stigma at HBCUs and in earlier educational environments, media, community, and even their own families, who are often fat themselves. There are even more administrative and academic campaigns that further stigmatize the higher-weight HBCU black students, faculty, and staff as the federally funded "war on obesity" (really a war on higher- and highest-weight people) are targeting HBCUs in particular and African Americans in general for their campaigns.

The HBCU Lincoln University in Pennsylvania at first began *requiring* all higher -weight students (30 or higher body mass index, almost all of them black *women*), including seniors who were expecting to graduate that semester, to take and pass a "Fitness for Life" class or forfeit their degrees. After a national uproar, the faculty voted to make the class a recommendation but not an additional requirement for graduation.[37] "James L. DeBoy, chair of Lincoln's health, physical education and recreation department, [was] . . . the most public proponent of the requirement. [DeBoy said,] "Any factor/trait/characteristic [i.e., their fatness] that we believe will hinder students' [mostly female, fat, black students] maximum development and full realization of life goals must be: (1) brought to their attention; (2) substantiated as being detrimental; and (3) adequately redressed."[38]

WHITE TRUMPS FAT FOR FEMALES

The "race-neutral" preference for fat women among men of color seems to exist only in some misinformed white people's perception of black and Latino culture. To comprehend the pain or even anger many black women feel when black men flirt with, date, and marry white women of any size requires understanding the intersectionalities of race, size, and gender in straight African American women's ability to get a date with a man of any race and at any weight, much less a committed relationship, husband, or soul mate.

More Americans than ever—87 percent—completely or somewhat agree that "it's all right for Blacks and Whites to date each other."[39] Yet straight black women have the fewest social options of all other race/gender dyads in the country. There are increasingly more black and brown men and women in the country.[40] In the United States, one in six new marriages is interracial, now only second in the world to Brazil.[41] However, black women are the *least* likely of any race or gender to get married at all.[42] Besides love, companionship, and 1,138 federal benefits,[43] marriage provides a plethora of mental and physical health, tax, and social benefits.[44] Most black women will never experience those benefits at all, or if they do, it will be for a relatively shorter time than other-race United Statesians.[45]

While black women are the least likely to marry in or out of their race, black men are the most likely men to marry out of their race.[46] I agree with Dr. Tiya Miles, an African American woman, MacArthur Fellowship "genius" grant recipient, and chair of the University of Michigan Afroamerican and African Studies Department, when she says that many black women feel hurt, demoralized, and even a little angry when they see a black man with a white woman.[47] Miles says the driving force behind her hurt feelings is her "awareness of all the [straight] African American women—beautiful, smart, good women, some of them [her] own family and friends—who might not have a honey to bring home this Thanksgiving holiday because they cannot find a date, even as rising numbers of eligible African American men will be wooing White women."[48]

Often fat acceptance organizations hold dances and other social events where the straight fat women are predominantly white. The black women present have to face the fewer black, fat-admiring men there fawning over mostly, or exclusively, the white women. That can make the fat acceptance event just another fat black woman rejection event. This is especially true if the white, male fat admirers are as neglectful of the black fat women as are the black men. In a perfect world love would be blind, but the racial hierarchy in the media and the broader culture dramatically influences dating and partnership behavior on multiple levels. One study found that more than 90 percent of the white men who express a racial preference prefer *not* to date only *one* type of woman—a *black woman*, no matter what she weighs.[49]

Researchers at the University of California–Irvine propose a "racial-beauty exchange theory." That is, "the notion that a [higher-weight] White woman who is less attractive by the measure of the dominant Euro-American beauty standard is willing to "trade down" on the racial hierarchy by dating a Black man. By the same token Black men who date ['even' higher-weight) White women are trading up" on the American racial hierarchy.[50] If higher-weight black women are already feeling devalued in their own communities (Many of us are.), social events at most size acceptance organizations may prove more of the same.

Another example of the difficulties African American women may have in fat activism leadership is when, also many years ago, a fat activism magazine editor sought me out to write a multipart series about the experience of fat black women. However, once I sent her the first two installments, the editor was not at all pleased to find that my article included much of the pain African American fat women go through because of our size in both the black and broader community.

She also questioned my authority to talk about my own psychological pain from fat discrimination because my doctorate was in communication, not psychology. If I recall correctly, the magazine editor/owner was a high school graduate and a self-taught editor and entrepreneur who had started the beautiful, slick fat activist magazine "from her kitchen table." So that fat woman's *white* privilege allowed her to call into question my credibility as a writer of my own life experience and researcher of others', even though I had far more training and experience in being black, fat, and me, much less writing and research.

When I asked the editor on what she based her notion that there was no discrimination against fat black women in the African American community, the editor said that on the way to her own white church every Sunday, she would see fat black women dressed in bright-colored hats and clothes smiling on their way to church. This was before online, and in larger cities brick-and-mortar, specialty shops that cater to large black women and offer ornate matching "Sunday-go-to-meeting" clothes and accessories. I told the editor that those women had probably made the clothes themselves and were happy because they were going to see someone who may have been the only man who didn't criticize them for their weight—the Lord . . . though the preacher and parishioners may.

That editor decided not to print any of the series she had solicited because my experience did not correlate with her notion of a happy land where fat black women danced free of size discrimination.

Though without fat-positive support, I remained interested in fat activism in my research and personal life because I found that weight stigma remained a central, painful, relevant issue in my life and in the media, my area of specialization as a university professor. As the "war on obesity" raged farther and wider, my ability to be taken seriously about ending weight stigma in the media and in my own life seemed to shrink.

A communication department colleague asked me to submit a paper to copresent on a Black Studies Division panel at a regional Popular Culture/American Culture Association (PCA/ACA) conference. He also alerted me to the PCA Fat Studies (FS) Division. At the conference I eagerly attended FS sessions seeking community and support. Unfortunately, I was the only African American at the FS sessions and the only one who spoke up when a younger, white, very thin graduate student espoused obviously white supremacist, poorly researched material.

A couple of white women looked at me sympathetically. A couple of others said a few supportive words to me briefly later in the day. But no one stood up for me in the session or stopped the white supremacist woman from her nasty retorts that what she said had to be true because she had found it on two websites (of zero credibility). I still held out hope for the larger *National* PCA/ACA conference. To my relief I found the national FS Division much more inclusive of women of color and other oppressed groups of differences (sexual orientation, transgender, etc.). Marilyn Wann, author, size acceptance movement star, and member of the National PCA FS Division, referred me to the Association for Size Diversity and Health. That association's biannual international educational conference proved a turning point in providing a sense of community and support that allowed me to fully reenter fat activism leadership.

STUMBLING BLOCKS INTO STEPPING-STONES

Langston Hughes's iconic Harlem Renaissance poem "Mother to Son" talks about how "Life ain't been no crystal stair"[51] for black women bearing the brunt of patriarchy and white supremacy while nurturing and supporting others, often with no one supporting them, in the climb we all must make. The poem also talks about how sometimes following our path means walking in darkness. Sometimes those dark places have never seen any light. Sometimes we have to make our own way and, without a pattern to follow, turn stumbling blocks into stepping-stones.

All of us working in fat activism know that it is difficult to make the time and find the resources to do the work. Few of us can afford to make this work our full-time endeavor because we have to earn a living. Most of us also have to use our hard-earned money to pay membership fees to fat activism organizations, pay our own way to conferences, purchase materials for conferences, and support fledgling public service activities that usually cost money far longer and more often than they ever turn a profit. Fat black women may have *even more difficulty* for a few reasons including but not limited to:

1. Fat black women are poorer and sicker. Thin women tend to make more money than fat women.[52] Eight out of 10 African American women are fat. African American women and Latinas earn less than all other race/gender groups in the country.[53] There is no statistical difference between African American women and Latinas across educational groups except at the master's degree level, where Latinas earn on average about $3,000 more than non-Latina, black women. Being poorer means a greater likelihood of being sicker without the money for preventative care and comforting interventions, much less critical health care.

2. It's more expensive for women to meet workplace dress codes and standards than it is for men.[54] It's *even more* expensive to be a black woman, especially when it comes to relaxing our hair or using wigs and weaves.[55] Though I personally find it worth the extra harassment, there can be hell to pay in our families as well as in the black and white communities if a black woman "chooses" to wear her unrelaxed, naturally kinky hair, including not getting hired or losing the job you have.[56]

3. Fat black women may be more stressed.[57] The multiple levels of discrimination fat black women face multiply the stress of each.

4. Fat black women are less likely to have a support system, more likely to be single head of household,[58] and more likely than any other race/gender category, perhaps by virtue of the Mammy stereotype, to be expected to happily care for others.[59] The Mammy stereotype began as a justification for slavery, later segregationist policies, and now the oppression of fat black women.[60] The Mammy is a higher-weight black woman, usually dark skinned and supposedly asexual and docile, who happily serves all the domestic needs of a white family with apparently none of her own.

Despite all these obstacles, I am not the only African American woman fat activism leader. There are a few who have beaten the odds and champion ending weight-based inequality specifically. There are more who challenge higher-weight discrimination as part of a broader context of ending all kinds of body and identity shaming, through fashion for higher-weight women. Maria Miranda, a fat black, Puerto Rican model for white fabric artist/fat women's fashion designer Rachel Kacenjar convinced me that fat women "having really kick-ass clothes" affirms those women and opens them up for fat activism political conscious raising in themselves and their audiences.[61]

Other women listed may just show up publically as their fabulous, sometimes fat, sometimes not, selves and behave in adipositive[62] ways in increasingly fat-hating culture. Here is an incomplete sampling of them in alphabetical order:

Jill Andrew and Felicia Fairclough are Afro-Canadian women who have a plus-size fashion blog called *Fat in the City*. Fairclough, a TV producer and program director for the Toronto International Body Image Film and Arts Festival, started *Fat in the City* to, "challenge size hatred b.s. through fashion."[63] Andrew is an "award-winning columnist, and international speaker on women and girls body image, self-esteem and empowerment."[64]

Sharon Baber, a self-described fat acceptance advocate, writes in her profanity-peppered blog *Nudemuse* about fat, race, sex, erotica, queer identities, as well as "body acceptance and challenging mainstream views of weight and the pitfalls of the diet and exercise industries."[65]

Collette Carter is codirector of the Audre Lorde Project (a community-organizing center for lesbian, gay, bisexual, two-spirit, trans, and gender nonconforming people of color) and a self-identified "black queer fat femme activist." She says, "I believe at the heart of lasting movement-building is the work of making spaces which help us sustain hope and the possibility for survival, as well as transformation."[66]

Stephanie Danforth produces the plus-size digital lifestyle magazine *Daily Venus Divas* whose mission is to give "plus size women a space to discuss fashion, dating, body image, and community issues."[67]

Etang Inyang and Tammy Johnson of Raks Africa, an Oakland, California, award-winning dancing duo, see belly dancing as a "necessary intervention for confronting body shamming and size policing ... working for body justice and the unity of people of every size."[68]

Ms. Vagina Jenkins is a higher-weight queer burlesque starlet who says her performances communicate the "message of challenging the traditional views of beauty" and increase visibility for the communities she represents, "women of size, people of color and queer femmes."[69]

Cassy Jones-McBryde is founder of the international Fuller Woman Network Expo. The Expo "is comprised of women all over the world [who] are committed to the mission of embracing who we are as women and creating a dialog of acceptance and celebration." She wants to help plus-size women celebrate and create body-positive images and events.[70]

Chenese Lewis was the first woman crowned Miss Plus America in 2003. She is a plus-size advocate whose podcast *The Chenese Lewis Show* was nominated for a People's Choice Award. She played a role in Monique's 2006 film

Phat Girls, and on January 6, 2014, *Ebony* magazine named her one of "6 Plus Fashion Power Players on the Rise."[71]

Naima Lowe and Galadriel Mozee are both signees of the NOLOSE (a fat and queer activism group) letter to the fat community about ways to end white supremacy in the fat activism movement in 2010.[72] At the time Mozee was copresident of NOLOSE. Mozee is a writer, and community educator, and has worked with the food justice movement for many years. Lowe describes herself as a fat, queer, African American artist and scholar.

Dr. Angela Denise Mensah, PhD, is an assistant professor of speech at the Eastern Campus of Cuyahoga Community College (Tri-C) in Cleveland, Ohio. Though not a fat activist per se and someone who believes no one group of people is more affected by oppression than any other, she does do research about body image in the African American community. She also looks at how weight stigma "complicates the life experience of some large and obese African American women."[73]

Miasia is a higher-weight, formally trained, professional Middle Eastern belly dancer who has performed for NOLOSE and internationally. Her goal as a teacher and performer is to open "the doorway of dance to include all bodies, sizes and abilities."[74]

Wendy O'Neal, perhaps not a fat activist per se, shows up as higher-weight African American woman, cultural worker, facilitator, and educator. She has been the keynote speaker for NOLOSE and "connects social and economic justice groups' mission, vision and values with how everyday work gets done ... She uses spiritually grounded practices, art, story circles and song sharing as tools for growing inspiration and sharing methodology for democratic process."[75]

Sonya Renee is a beautiful, bald, Baltimorean fat woman, former National Individual Poetry Slam Champion, and founder of The Body Is Not an Apology. Her online movement promotes "radical self-love (as) the foundation for radical human love, and therefore a vehicle to social justice."[76] In addition to facing the sizeism, Renee is a dark-skinned woman who also must battle white supremacist colorism that values lighter-skinned people, women in particular.

For icing on this triple-layered cake of courage, Renee sometimes is even courageous enough to perform publically with her (because of a childhood condition that made her kinky hair fall out) naturally bald head. Most black women who have naturally kinky or even curly hair usually wear straight-at-the-root wigs, weaves, or chemically relax their hair. White supremacist values pressure most black women into investing more money than they can afford and more internalized stigmatization than is healthy for them on wigs, weaves, and relaxers.[77]

Though 40 percent of those who are bald in the United States are women, most wear wigs.[78] Bald-headedness is another state stigmatized much more for women than men in mainstream patriarchal society. In the black community, even women who have very short hair are pejoratively called "bald-headed."

Kathryn Seabron, aka Juicy D. Light, is "founder and artistic director of *The Bodacious Bawdies,* an ethnically diverse large-size troupe with a focus on utilizing dance to range from joyful expression to activist acts."[79]

Miz Ginger Snapz, a higher-weight woman "who self-identifies as one of the country's Queer Black Burlesque Starlets," is part of a Baltimore city collective called the Charm City Kitty Club.[80] She says she is dedicated to promoting a diversity of sexualities, races, and bodies on stage and "committed to creating and maintaining an atmosphere free from racism, classism, ageism, ableism, biphobia, transphobia, homophobia, misogyny, cultural appropriation and censorship."

Lisa Tealer, a former aerobics instructor and health club owner, is a board member and director of programs for the National Association to Advance Fat Acceptance.[81] Since 1969, the association has been "a non-profit civil rights organization dedicated to ending size discrimination in all of its forms . . . [helping to] build a society in which people of every size are accepted with dignity and equality in all aspects of life . . . [and pursuing] this goal through advocacy, public education, and support."[82] Tealer says she wants more African American women in the size acceptance movement. **Phyllis Warr** is also a member of association's board, serving as membership services director.[83]

Bianca D. M. Wilson is the UCLA Williams Institute of Law Senior Scholar of Public Policy, NOLOSE (started out as the National Organization for Lesbians of SizE and are now open to fat queer equity and all allies)[84] fat activist, and a *Fat Studies Reader* author.

Jessica Wilson, MS, is a registered dietician who focuses on mindful or intuitive eating and believes that health and weight are not connected. She is active in Association for Size Diversity and Health and lives as a queer lower-weight woman on the West Coast.[85]

WHAT WHITE FAT ACTIVISTS CAN DO

White fat activists can also help women of color in the movement by "doing the work of learning about the histories and impacts of colonization and oppression on people of color . . . and allowing people's firsthand experiences of racism to be the final and authoritative voice on the subject of impact to communities of color," and following the other advice in the NOLOSE "A Response to White Fat Activism from People of Color in the Fat Justice Movement" letter.[86]

They can make sure that at social events men of all races treat black straight women with the same deference as they do white straight women. They can join white fabric artist/fat fashion designer Rachel Kacenjar and other moderators on the Anti Racism Resource Group for Size Activists Facebook page whose goal is for white people to "further and continue our learning and understanding about intentional and unintentional racism, systemic, and interpersonal racism and their effects on our activism ... to share resources and learn from each other ... [in an online] space that is intended as a place for White people and people with White privilege to work on [their] privilege & racism ... [where] all folks are welcome, but there is likely to be white/privileged processing and working through shit."[87] For a beginning that'll do. That'll do quite well. As for the black women already working in fat activism leadership: take to heart that Langston Hughes poem "Mother to Son."[88] That mother advises her son to be persistent in climbing the perilous stairway of life. No matter how hard it gets, keep going. Be comforted that you are indeed not alone in the journey. Look out for those of us like you are still fighting the good fight. Let us help bear one another's burdens and thereby halve them for each of us.

NOTES

1. Joel Whitburn, *Top R&B/Hip-Hop Singles: 1942–2004* (Menomonee Falls, WI: Record Research, 2004), 275.

2. Slone Epidemiological Center, "Black Women's Health Study," http://www.bu.edu/bwhs/.

3. Black Women's Health Study at Boston University, "Research Team," http://www.bu.edu/bwhs/research-team/.

4. Rochelle Zimmerman, "Why Are 4 Out of 5 Black Women Obese, Overweight?," *Common Health*, November 29, 2012, http://www.commonhealth.wbur.org/2012/11/why-are-four-out-of-five-black-women-obese.

5. Sadie Dingfelder, "African American Women at Risk," *American Psychological Association Monitor* 44, no. 1 (January 2013): 56.

6. Langston Hughes, "Mother to Son," in *Selected Poems of Langston Hughes* (New York: Random House, 1990), 187.

7. Lee Mun Wah, *The Color of Fear*, Stir Fry Seminars, 1994.

8. Zimmerman, "Why Are 4 out of 5 Black Women Obese, Overweight?"

9. Food Research and Action Center, "Overweight and Obesity in the U.S.," http://frac.org/initiatives/hunder-and-obesity/obesity-in-the-us/.

10. Mary Story et al., "The Epidemic of Obesity in American Indian Communities and the Need for Childhood Obesity-Prevention Programs," *American Journal of Clinical Nutrition* 69, no. 4 (April 1999): 747S–54S, http://ajcn.nutrition.org/content/69/4/747S.long#sec-3.

11. Centers for Disease Control, *Summary Health Statistics for U.S. Adults: National Health Interview Survey 2010*, table 31, p. 106, http://www.cdc.gov/nchs/data/series/sr _10/sr10_252.pdf.

12. Food Research and Action Center, "Overweight and Obesity in the U.S."

13. Mary Pipher, *Reviving Ophelia: Saving the Selves of Adolescent Girls* (Northampton, MA: Media Education Foundation Video Resources for the 21st Century, 2000).

14. Natalie Digate Muth, "What Are the Guidelines for Percentage of Body Fat Loss?," American Council on Exercise, Healthy Living: Fit Life, December 2, 2009, http://www.acefitness.org/acefit/healthy-living-article/60/112/what-are-the-guidelines -for-percentage-of/.

15. "Hispanic vs. Latino," Diffen, http://www.diffen.com/difference/Hispanic_vs _Latino.

16. Marilyn Glenville, "How to Lose Weight Naturally," 2012, http://www .marilynglenville.com/womens-health-issues/weight-control/.

17. Hermine H. Mayes, Michael C. Neale, and Linden J. Eaves, "Genetic and Environmental Factors in Relative Body Weight and Human Adiposity," *Behavioral Genetics* 4 (July 1997): 325.

18. Sandra Aasmodt, "Why Dieting Usually Doesn't Work," Ted Talks, 'http:// www.ted.com/talks/sandra_aamodt_why_dieting_usually_doesn't_work.html.

19. Jesse D. McKinnon and Claudette E. Bennet, "Black Population by Sex, 2000," in *We the People: Blacks in the United States, Census 2000 Special Reports* (Washington, DC: U.S. Census Bureau, August 2005), 1.

20. Michelle A. Vu, "African Americans Most Religiously Devout Group," *Christian Post*, February 2, 2009, http://www.christianpost.com/news/african -americans-most-religiously-devout-group-36736/.

21. Charles H. Lippy, ed., "Religious Issues Today: Dieting and Diet," in chap. 5, "Fundamentalism and Pentecostalism: The Changing Face of Evangelism Today," *Faith in America: Changes, Challenges, New Direction* (Santa Barbara, CA: ABC-CLIO), 1: 220.

22. Deb Burgard, "What Is 'Health at Every Size'?," in *The Fat Studies Reader*, ed. Esther Rothblum and Sondra Solovay (New York: New York University Press, 2009), 42–49.

23. *The Thistle*, "But Some of Us Are Brave: A History of Black Feminism in the United States," http://www.mit.edu/~thistle/v9/9.01/6blackf.html. "*The Thistle* is a now-defunct publication dedicated to human rights work on the Massachusetts Institute of Technology campus and across the globe, advocating for sexual assault awareness, gender and racial equality, and the elimination of MIT's support of apart-heid and genocide in Africa in the 1990s. As one can expect, it was unpopular with many in the upper tiers of MIT administration and now no longer exists as an active student group" (November 30, 2011, http://wiki.mitadmissions.org/The_Thistle).

24. Based on, "Myths That Divert Black Women from Our Own Freedom," in *The Thistle*, "But Some of Us Are Brave."

25. *Trickster at the Crossroads: West Africa's God of Messages, Sex and Deceit*, http:// www.techgnosis.com/chunkshow-single.php?chunk=chunkfrom-2005-06-15-2009-0.txt.

26. Don't see: Andrea Elizabeth Shaw, *The Embodiment of Disobedience: Fat Black Women's Unruly Political Bodies* (Lanham, MD: Lexington Books, 2006).

27. Brande Victorian, "Why do We Feel the Need to Keep Explaining 'Our' Fatness?," *MadameNoire.com – Black Women's Lifestyle*, May 7, 2012, http://badamenoire.comblackwomenslifestyle/174721/why-do-we-feel-the-need-to-keep-explaining-our-fatness/.

28. Ibid.

29. I am scheduled to do a presentation on the methodological flaws of studies who purport to support the hypothesis that black women experience no weight stigma, bullying, harassment, or psychological effect at the April 2014 National Popular Culture/American Culture Conference in Chicago.

30. Stephanie Covington Armstrong, "Room for Debate: One Size Does Not Fit All," *New York Times*, February 13, 2013, http://www.nytimes.com/roomfordebate/2012/05/07/women-weight-and-wellness/one-size-does-not-fit-all-8nytimes.com.

31. Just one of many such studies: Anita Simmons, "Black Womanhood, Misogyny, and Hip-Hop Culture: A Feminist Intervention," *Cultural Landscapes* 1, no. 2 (2008): 27–48.

32. Tiya Miles, "Black Women, Interracial Dating, and Marriage: What's Love Got to Do with It?," Huff Post: BLACKVOICES, November 5, 2013, http://www.huffingtonpost.com/tiya-miles/interracial-dating-and-marriage_b_4213066.html.

33. Amber Sutton, "Alabama State University's Plus-Size Dance Team to Perform on Steve Harvey Show May 31" (video), Al.com, http://www.al.com/entertainment/index.ssf/2013/05/alabama_state_universitys_plus.html.

34. Ibid.

35. Terry Manning, "Meet the Honey Beez," *Montgomery Advertiser*, http://www.montgomeryadvertiser.com/VideoNetwork/2224226585001/Meet-the-Honeybeez.

36. Ernie Suggs, "Males a Definite Minority at HBCUs," ajc.com, February 1, 2012, http://www.ajc.com/news/news/local/males-a-distinct-minority-at-hbcus/nQQqT/.

37. Scott Jaschic, "Lincoln U. Ends Obesity Rule," *Inside Higher Education*, http://www.insidehighered.com/news/2009/12/07/lincoln.

38. Ibid.

39. Pew Research Center for the People and the Press, "Section 1: How Generations Have Changed: Generations, Social Issues and Religion," November 3, 2011, p. 7, http://www.people-press.org/2011/11/03/the-generation-gap-and-the-2012-election-3/11-3-11-20/.

40. Pew Research Center for the People and the Press, "Nation's Race & Ethnicity in 2011: % by Generation," p. 2.

41. Linsey Davis and Eric Noll, "Interracial Marriage More Common than Ever, but Black Women Still Lag," ABC News, June 4, 2010, http://abcnews.go.com?WN/Media/black-women-marry-interracial-marriage-common/story?id=10830719.

42. Ibid.

43. Jacob Silverman, "How Marriage Works: Benefits of Marriage," http://people.howstuffworks.com/marriage1.htm.

44. United States Conference of Catholic Bishops, "What Are the Social Benefits of Marriage?," For Your Marriage, http://www.foryourmarriage.org/what-are-the-social-benefits-of-marriage/.

45. Rose M. Kreider, "Remarriage in the United States," poster presented at the annual meeting of the American Sociological Association, Montreal, August 10–14, 2006, 9, citing the U.S. Census Bureau, "Survey of Income and Program Participation, 1996, 2001 and 2004 Panels, Wave 2."

46. Ibid.

47. Alexis Garrett Stodghill, "Interracial Marriage and Single Black Women: African American Dating Issues Come Home for the Holiday," The Grio, November 6, 2013, http://www.thegrio.com/2013/11/06/interracial-dating-marriage -love-black-men-women-white-native-american/; and Miles, "Black Women, Interracial Dating, and Marriage."

48. Miles, "Black Women, Interracial Dating, and Marriage."

49. The University of Irvine scholars Cynthia Feliciano, Belinda Robnett, and Golnaz Komaie have requested researchers NOT to cite without permission the online draft of a paper that they prepared for presentation at the Population Association of America 2008 annual meeting, Session 171, New Orleans, LA, April 19, 2008. Permission requested January 2014. At press permission is still pending, so no specific citation is made.

50. As discussed in Miles, "Black Women, Interracial Dating, and Marriage."

51. Hughes, "Mother to Son."

52. Timothy A. Judge, Charlice Hurst, and Lauren S. Simon, "Does It Pay to Be Smart, Attractive, or Confident (or All Three)?: Relationships among General Mental Ability, Physical Attractiveness, Core Self-Evaluations, and Income," *Journal of Applied Psychology* 94, no. 3 (2009): 747.

53. U.S. Census Bureau, "Table 8: Mean Income in 2004 by Educational Attainment of Population 18 Years and Older by Age, Sex, Race Alone, and Hispanic Origin 2005," *Current Population Survey 2005 Annual Social and Economic Supplement*, October 26, 2006.

54. Rebecca Adams, "That Is Why It Is More Expensive to Be a Woman," *Huffington Post*, http://www.huffingtonpost.com/2013/09/23/beauty-products_n _3975209.html.

55. H. Fields Grenee, "What Spending Half a Trillion Dollars on Hair Care and Weaves Says about Us," Madame Noire, May 11, 2011, http://madamenoire.com/ 57134/what-spending-a-half-a-trillion-dollars-on-hair-care-and-weaves-says-about-us/.

56. There are many reports of this type. For one of the latest examples, see Julee Wilson, "Black Executive Allegedly Fired for Braided Hair and Ethnic Clothing," Huff Post: Black Voices, December 9, 2013, http://www.huffingtonrpost.com/2013/ 12/09/black-executive-fired-bp-hair-ethnic-clothing-_n_4413543.html.

57. Arline T. Geronimus et al., "Do US Black Women Experience Stress-Related Accelerated Biological Aging?: A Novel Theory and First Population-Based Test of Black-White Differences in Telomere Length," *Human Natural Margins* 21, no. 1 (March 10, 2010): 19–38, http://www.ncbi.nlm.nih.gov/pmc/articles/ PMC2861506/.

58. U.S. Department of Health and Human Services, Health Resources and Services Administration, Maternal and Child Health Bureau, Women's Health USA

2012 (Rockville, MD: U.S. Department of Health and Human Services, 2013), http://www.mchb.hrsa.gov/whusa12/pc/pages/hc.html.

59. Enid Vàzquez, "Everyone Needs a Support System," *Positively Aware*, September/October 2012, http://positivelyaware.com/2012/12_06/everyone-needs-a-support-system.shtml.

60. Melissa V. Harris-Perry, *Sister Citizen: Shame, Stereotypes, and Black Women in America* (New Haven, CT: Yale University Press), 72.; Terri M. Adams and Douglas B. Fuller, "The Words Have Changed but the Ideology Remains the Same: Misogynistic Lyrics in Rap Music," *Journal of Black Studies* 36, no. 6 (July 2006): 994.

61. Chris Miller, *The Balance of Fashion: The Art of Rachel Kacenjar*, March 11, 2013, http://www.youtube.com/watch?v=sa5JbEcMdR0.

62. Substantia Jones, "The Adipositive Project," http://adipositivity.com/.

63. Fat in the City—Curvy Plus Size Fashion Blog, "About Fat in the City," http://www.fatinthecity.com/about.

64. Fat in the City—Curvy Plus Size Fashion Blog, "Mission Statement," http://www.fatinthecity.com/about.

65. Jennée Desmond-Harris, "Black Obesity: Shannon Barber and Fat Acceptance," The Root, May 2012, http://www.theroot.com/articles/culture/2012/05/black_obesity_shannon_barber_and_fat_acceptance.html.

66. NOLOSE, "2012 Fat Strikes Back! Keynote Speaker," http://nolose.org/12/.

67. *Ebony* magazine, "Curvy Plus: 6 Fashion Power Players on the Rise," January 6, 2014, http://www.ebony.com/photos/style/curvy-plus-6-fashion-power-players-on-the-rise-405#axzz301KCE0ZH.

68. "Your Body Raks," Facebook.

69. Diana Bagby, "Queer Burlesque Performer Vagina Jenkins Seeks International Fame," The GA Voice, April 1, 2010, http://www.thegavoice.com/aae/nightlife/119-queer-burlesque-performer-vagina-jenkins-seeks-international-fame.

70. *Ebony* magazine, "Curvy Plus."

71. Ibid.

72. Tara Shuai et al., "A Response to White Fat Activism from People of Color in the Fat Justice Movement," NOLOSE: The Revolution Just Got Bigger, 2010, http://www.nolose.org/activism/POC.php.

73. Angels Denise Mensah, "The Fat 'Other,' " Binge Eating Disorder Association: Weight Stigma in Diverse Populations, September 8, 2013, http://bedaonline.com/wsaw2013/weight-stigma-diverse-populations-angela-mensah-phd/#.Ut3derRMHIU.

74. NOLOSE, "2010 Performance!: Miasia," http://nolose.org/10/performance.php.

75. NOLOSE, "Bridge to Fatlandia: Exploring Citizenship while Bravely Building Fat Pride Community," http://nolose.org/10/.

76. Liz Harby, "Local Artists: Sonya Renee," http://whatweekly.com/2012/09/20/sonya-renee-taylor/.

77. Fields Grenee, "What Spending Half a Trillion Dollars."

78. See "Female Beauty and the Sociology of Stigma," The Rachel Tanner Memorial Prize for Visual Sociology, Social Science Research Council, 2013, http://www.racheltanurmemorialprize.org/female-beauty-and-the-sociology-of-stigma/; and

Kathryn Coe et al., "The Enigma of the Stigma of Hair Loss: Why Is Cancer-Treatment Related Alopecia so Traumatic for Women?," *The Open Cancer Journal* 6 (2013): 1–8, http://www.benthamscience.com/open/tocj/articles/V006/1TOCJ.pdf.

79. NOLOSE, "2010 Presenter Bios: Kathryn Seabron," http://nolose.org/10/performance.php.

80. Charm City Kitty Club, "Fun from the Fall 2013 Breakup Show," http://charmcitykittyclub.wordpress.com/tag/miz-ginger-snapz/.

81. Lisa Tealer, "Enough with the Stereotypes of Fat and Thin People," May 8, 2012, http://www.nytimes.com/roomfordebate/2012/05/07/women-weight-and-wellness/enough-with-the-stereotypes-of-fat-article.

82. "Welcome to NAAFA.org," http://www.naafaonline.com/dev2/.

83. "Board Members, Board of Directors," http://www.naafaonline.com/dev2/about/Board.html.

84. "NOLOSE: All Genders, with a Shared Ideology," NOLOSE: WHO WE ARE, http://www.nolose.org/11/genderpolicy.php.

85. Jessica Wilson, My *Kitchen Dietitian*, http://mykitchendietitian.com/blog/about/.

86. Shuai et al., "A Response to White Fat Activism."

87. Rachel Kacenjar, "Hey Newbies, Please Read Our Community Guidelines," Facebook: Anti-Racism Resource Group for Size Activists.

88. Hughes, "Mother to Son."

17

Cows, Pigs, Whales: Nonhuman Animals, Antifat Bias, and Exceptionalist Logics

Kristen A. Hardy

In the context of social justice work, it is common for proponents of specific causes to find themselves in conflict with others whose commitments are centered in a different variety of equity-related advocacy. For example, prodiversity activists may be challenged by feminist projects that address culturally specific forms of female oppression, while some women's rights advocates may bristle at the defense of cultural or religious practices that appear to them to be less than equitable. Lesbian, gay, bisexual, and transgender advocates often embrace and celebrate notions of sexuality and gender identity that appear essentialist from some feminist theoretical positions, while efforts by the latter to deconstruct identity categories may be viewed as a threat to self-conceptions considered empowering by queer or transgender individuals and groups. Those involved in antipoverty efforts may take issue with attempts to "fracture" solidarity by addressing racism, sexism, homophobia, and other forms of bias within class-oriented advocacy work, while dispossessed persons who are also marginalized on the basis of other social identities often insist that differential needs and experiences be recognized within socioeconomic categories.

This type of "intercause" conflicts is a frequent occurrence for those seeking to raise awareness within human-oriented advocacy communities of the exploitation faced by nonhuman animals. A reluctance on the part of many social movements to even entertain the inclusion of animal rights within their existing mandates presents a major challenge to animal advocates who seek to integrate their causes within a broader network of progressive efforts. In order to effectively address this issue, however, it is necessary to examine the larger context and deeper underpinnings of this division. How may persons who are committed to equity-related work, but who also reject the "exceptionalist" position that there is some clear, universal, definitive distinction between humans and other animals, negotiate the fraught relationship between "human rights" and "animal rights"?

Among the most significant theoretical developments in late-twentieth-century social justice circles was that of intersectionality. Arising in the context of feminism and critical race studies, the term has its origins in the work of legal scholar Kimberlé Crenshaw, who aimed to better capture the complex position of women of color vis-à-vis existing discourses on race and gender by "contrast[ing] the multidimensionality of Black women's experience with the single-axis analysis that distorts these experiences."[1]

In the years following Crenshaw's pioneering contribution, the concept of intersectionality has entered into a variety of disciplines, primarily in the social sciences, to become a much-used theoretical tool for the study of historical and contemporary forms of inequity.[2] While, as Jennifer C. Nash writes, "intersectionality invites scholars to come to terms with the legacy of exclusions of multiply marginalized subjects from feminist and anti-racist work, and the impact of those absences on both theory and practice,"[3] the scope of subject positions considered by intersectional analyses also continues to expand beyond race and gender, to embrace class, sexuality, gender identity, disability, age, and other salient social categories. Further, the notion of approaching oppression as a matrix—a system in which any given variety of marginalization is dependent on an entire network of interrelated biases and privileges—has opened up fruitful new avenues for many varieties of social justice-oriented work, both inside and outside of academia. For example, a sociologist working from an intersectional perspective might examine how hierarchical constructions of gender that devalue women are interconnected with homophobic perceptions of male "effeminacy" and powerful heterocentric cultural narratives of masculinity.[4] Similarly, understanding the roles of socioeconomic class and gender in shaping disabled individuals' experiences depends on an intersectional conception of social identity.[5] This type of approach has contributed not only to forging new avenues of intellectual understanding but also to generating intensified calls for cooperative antioppressive work among adherents of various social movements.

For those scholars and activists whose critical perspective extends to the questioning of conventional distinctions and boundaries between humans and nonhuman animals, the absence of such concerns within conventional social justice circles is often acutely felt, especially within analyses and advocacy that are otherwise resolutely intersectional. Some work has begun to appear in the margins of existing academic fields, seeking to introduce nonhuman participants into the purview of critical scholarship. Ecofeminism is notable in this regard, with its adoption of an "ecological" model for studying networks of interdependencies that cross the nature/culture divide.[6] Also,

within the emergent field of critical animal studies, a few pioneering researchers have started to explicitly address concerns that could be regarded as intersectional in nature, such as the relations between marginalization of
nonhuman animals and women of color,[7] and the affinity of animal rights
and disability self-advocacy.[8]

Yet more-mainstream and better-established traditions of research and
activism have often been reluctant to introduce this sort of porosity into the
boundaries of their conventionally human-oriented perspectives. Among the
best-known attempts to seriously address some of these concerns in a critical
and sustained fashion are those of noted theorist Donna Haraway, whose
recent work has introduced the nature and ethics of interspecies relations as
viable topics for discussion among a broader academic audience.[9] Yet in spite
of such efforts, there remains a gulf between animal advocacy circles and many
human-oriented equity movements, as well as between their allied fields of
scholarship. Indeed, the frequent use of "social justice" and "human rights"
as if these terms were unproblematically synonymous testifies to the tenacity
of anthropocentrism within the social sciences and social activist spheres,
and, in turn, to the difficulties faced by critical animal scholars and animal
advocates in making inroads within these communities.

Academics and activists with human rights commitments often articulate
critique and resistance to prejudice and discrimination by framing the core
concern as one of "dehumanization." Critics of racism, sexism, classism, dis/
ableism, and other forms of prejudice frequently call upon the view that the
fundamental mechanism—and ultimate effect—of such systemic biases is the
denial of full humanity to members of the particular group(s) at issue.[10]
Indeed, historical and contemporary bodies of discourse and imagery lend
strong support to the idea that removing traditional physical and/or cultural
markers of human status and, frequently, replacing them with characteristics
ascribed to nonhumans has long been a prevalent method of marking members of particular groups as inferior. The consequences, depending on purpose
and context, have ranged from ridicule to genocide.

Rarely, however, is much attention given to exploring the anthropocentric
assumptions that underlie this particular framing. The practice of representing
"other-ed" individuals and groups as lacking in or devoid of humanity, in at
least some respects, is undoubtedly a central one in the perpetuation of bias.
Yet when this recognition is carried over from the level of *description* of such
representations and adopted as a point of *critique* of the social justice implications thereof, there is a danger of overlooking the deeper and more problematic implications of the concept itself. For "dehumanization" to even be an
intelligible idea, there must exist an underlying hierarchy in which human
and nonhuman differences are understood as meaningful criteria of evaluation
against universal, trans-species norms and ideals. We might do well to ask

what sorts of ontologies or "ways of being" are reinforced when we frame our critique of biased representations through a lens that itself uncritically accepts the notion that to be portrayed as "other than human" is automatically to be reduced to a state of lesser being.

In this chapter, I question the idea that we can ever truly treat the concept of "dehumanization" purely as a self-evident entity—as solely *figurative* in meaning, a mere synonym for denigration or degradation, divorced from its deeper implications. This is particularly a concern since the categories of humanity and animality referenced by "dehumanization" are, arguably, core structuring elements of Western thought and therefore at the heart of the matrix of interlinked oppressions. If we, as critical scholars, wish to advocate for the consideration of the place of nonhuman beings within systems of power, we cannot afford to ignore the full implications of the tools that are deployed in analyzing and resisting exploitation and domination of humans.

In examining this issue, I have chosen to address a specific pair of equity-oriented academic/activist movements within which I am also a participant: critical fat studies and fat acceptance.[11] The discourses of analysis and resistance articulated by these movements are among the places where one may find the identification and refutation of "dehumanization" embraced as an important part of questioning the assumptions, biases, and discriminatory practices around fatness and fat persons. Yet, I argue, for all its evident advantages, "dehumanization" remains a problematic element of critique—one that not only contributes to the continued oppression of nonhumans but also acts to subtly undermine the very possibility of a more equitable condition for all human beings, as sought by these and similar social justice projects.

I will begin by briefly exploring the nature of the conventional distancing of the human from the nonhuman in Western thought and consider why the concept of "dehumanization" holds enduring interest within human rights and equity contexts. Then, through examining cultural practices of representing fat subjects, I will reflect upon why naming and criticizing dehumanization is found to be a useful strategy by many body diversity activists and scholars. Finally, I shall briefly consider some alternative possibilities for rethinking fat activism and animal rights that are mindful of underlying intersectional concerns.

Categories are never innocent but always bear traces the power relations out of which they emerge. From the time of Aristotle onward, Western philosophers have grappled with the origin and role of the concepts, classes, and taxonomies according to which we organize, engage with, and attempt to explain the world. In more recent times, social scientists have also involved themselves in this quest; while often disagreeing over whether to preserve or deconstruct those categories into which social actors are sorted, few would deny that they provide an essential lens onto the ways in which social groups and communities evaluate, sort, and demarcate their members.[12]

Of particular concern to scholars of human-nonhuman relations are the historical and contemporary practices by which Western culture delineates *Homo sapiens* from all other animal species collectively, and, in turn, the processes by which this boundary has been made into one of the most fundamental organizing principles of modernity. Some authors who align themselves with critical animal studies have engaged directly with specific aspects of this issue,[13] as have various others, including scholars of history,[14] philosophy,[15] and geography.[16] However, even when not explicitly brought to the fore, the question of what, if anything, makes humans deserving of "exceptional" status within the animal world—and how claims to this effect have shaped our worldviews, our relationships, our institutions, and our practices—nevertheless remains at issue.

Discussions of rights, human or otherwise, often invoke the legal language of "personhood." However, this dimension is only one of many grounds upon which such determinations are made in everyday practice. Evaluating—whether formally or informally, consciously or not—the extent to which a given individual or group is "owed" inclusion within a given sphere of rights, freedoms, or community hinges upon a broader consideration: how fully "human" the subject in question is deemed to be.

To take an extended and somewhat oblique approach to defining "humanity" for the purposes of this study, let us begin by questioning what it means, within a modern Western worldview, to be included within the category of "the human." By focusing upon a number of what may be thought of as *axes of inclusion and exclusion*, we can establish a skeleton for ordering and analyzing some of the key elements of widely shared assumptions about humanity. These criteria, even when merely implicit, have functioned as powerful forces to exclude certain individuals and groups according to an underlying logic that continues to deeply impact Euro-American thought about the world and its inhabitants.

Firstly, to identify someone as "human" strongly implies *social* inclusion. Conventionally, when one is considered to exist within the realm of the social, we assume his or her participation as a social actor within a network of human relationships. The human subject, in traditional sociological thought, is framed as capable of choosing to act in ways that contribute to societal progress, order, and cohesion—or, in some cases, to their opposites. He or she is understood as a distinct individual who may partake in any of a range of social identities that integrate him or her into the broader social networks that collectively compose the social world.

Indeed, while it has long been recognized by biologists and zoologists that nonhuman animals inhabit societies made up of their own species mates as well as members of other species, there has been resistance within the social sciences to acknowledging the "multispecies" character of what we think of as "human" society and to recognizing that nonhuman animals are indispensable "social actors" within human social institutions in ways that have varied across time and space. This failure to take into account the social statuses and roles of nonhumans—a consequence of a worldview that takes human-only boundaries of our social world as a largely unquestioned norm—has led to the formulation of academic disciplines that artificially circumscribe human experience and behavior and misleadingly separate human beings from the broader contexts of their social existence. Only relatively recently have the social sciences seen the emergence of a significant collection of meaningful attempts to reweave our ideas about the social realm in ways that recognize the entanglement of other species with ourselves.[17]

Secondly, to be recognized as a human being entails a *cultural* inclusion, a participation in a sphere of symbolic meaning making. Traditionally the domain of anthropological study, culture has long been regarded as both the exclusive possession and the essential marker of the *anthropos*—indeed, many contemporary sources continue to define "culture" specifically in terms of humans' ability to surpass the given conditions of their natural environment.[18]

An exceedingly fluid concept, conventional academic usage has commonly linked culture intimately with communication, particularly the creation of shared bodies of experience and knowledge.[19] While this aspect of culture is not inherently species-exclusionary, when situated within a framework of dominant Euro-American assumptions, beliefs, and norms about language, it quite easily becomes read as such. For example, the capability to both "speak" and "respond"—to communicate in an interactive fashion, acknowledging the words and actions of others and intelligently engaging therewith—has long been considered the hallmark of human communication patterns. However, the long history of scientists' resistance to including complex forms of nonhuman communication within the boundaries of "language"[20] has contributed to the constitution of "culture" as a human-only entity.

Not only is "culture" traditionally set apart in discourse from "nature," but it has tended to be set *against* the latter.[21] In defining "cultural" aspects of life as those that supersede what is thought to simply exist unaltered by human minds and hands is to define "nature" itself as the passive raw material through which human beings achieve their distinctive "humanness." From this perspective, "the natural" becomes the less-valued residual category to which all nonhuman life is consigned; in contrast, partaking in "the cultural" marks the human as capable of transcendence of nature. As many feminist scholars have pointed out, the "nature" that is thereby surpassed has included, in many contexts, the physical body (especially the female body), viewed as inherently tainted by its own inherently "fleshy" biological character.[22]

Closely linked to culture is what we might term *religio-ethical* inclusion. Particularly in the Christian tradition, though not confined exclusively to it, notions of a moral life are closely bound up with discourses of self-discipline, restraint, and austerity.

Such values and aspirations are not inherently opposed to a positive acknowledgment of humans' continuity with the nonhuman world—one need only consider, for example, the importance of these and similar values in traditions such as Hinduism, Buddhism, Jainism, Sikhism, or Taoism, which have each set forth a worldview that professes a significant degree of metaphysical interrelatedness or "interbeing" among humans and nonhuman species.[23] This positive emphasis is also not entirely absent from Western traditions; from the well-known writings of Francis of Assisi (1182–1226) to the more-modern "nature mysticism" of figures like Ralph Waldo Emerson (1803–82) and Henry David Thoreau (1817–62), strands of spiritual thought have repeatedly arisen that combine religiously grounded or Christian-inflected ethics with a more open attitude toward interspecies community and communion.

However, such attitudes have often been eclipsed by more forthrightly exceptionalist views of the human subject within Western religious thought. From theological arguments for human ensoulment alone, to attempts at biblical justification of "Man's" dominion—often sliding into de facto domination—over all of nature, much of mainstream Christian thinking, including that of prominent Christian theologians like Thomas Aquinas (1225–74) as well as foundational Protestant figures like Martin Luther (1483–1546) and John Calvin (1509–64), has maintained a clear and distinct human-nonhuman hierarchical relationship.[24] Within a framework that casts the "physical" in opposition to the "spiritual," the association of the morally good subject with the self-controlled individual has often fostered an orientation toward the body, and, more broadly, toward the nonhuman "natural" world, as a sphere of unruly physicality to be bridled and overcome.[25]

Also relevant here is *philosophical* inclusion. Western philosophy, in its conventional formulations from the Greeks through to contemporary times, has tended to center the human—and often, implicitly or otherwise, the *male* human specifically—both as the source of meaning, values, and logic within the world, and as the principal object of philosophical reflection and debate. While the question of the nature of "the animal" has been a reoccurring one for philosophers, ancient and modern, much of the work on this topic has revolved around the identification of specific qualities and capacities of human uniqueness vis-à-vis the nonhuman occupants of the world,[26] or, somewhat more progressively, the crafting of an ethic for humans' treatment of nonhumans.[27]

Such considerations, however, have only rarely moved on to engage critically with the more fundamental questions underlying humans' assertions of their exceptional status within the spectrum of living beings. Indeed, Western traditions of secular thought have, for the most part, structured the very delineation of who counts as a "subject," who possesses agency, and who is capable of exercising reason, along a human-nonhuman axis, relegating other animals to the position of "the other" against whom "humanness" is itself defined.[28] It may be argued that from such a perspective the nonhuman animal exists always in a state of, at best, limited and highly constrained subjectivity.

The *political* is another important terrain of inclusion and exclusion. In virtually every manifestation of political theorizing, it is humans alone—and, commonly, only a subset thereof—who are granted the right to participate in the *polis* as full citizens. Not merely a question of enfranchisement, citizenship entails access to an array of rights and freedoms that are often granted incompletely, if at all, to the noncitizen. As a full and documented member of a contemporary nation-state, the citizen partakes in a national identity that grants him or her a recognized political status and, paradoxically, at least some degree of protection from domination by the state itself.[29]

Further, within the modern system of biopolitical and neoliberal governance, the legitimate citizen, to whom the benefits of the state are owed, is one who has been *responsibilized*–that is, who actively takes measures to ensure his or her own welfare, including adherence to those norms deemed conducive to a certain vision of the collective good.[30] In taking on the role of the self-regulating subject, the individual is cast as a socially and morally competent citizen.

Closely linked with the political dimension, we may point to *economic* inclusion as another significant axis. Within the structure of late capitalism, the labor of those classed as nonhuman remains a core component of production and exchange. But such labor is often made "invisible" or, at least, framed as legitimate for exploitation without compensation, beyond, at most, the bare sustenance of life—and then too, only while the laboring body is considered to be maximally productive for the benefit of those who are deemed fully human and fully citizen.[31]

The "excluded" class who is granted little to no claim to the economic fruits of their own labors has extended to a variety of communities during various periods in the modern era, including black Africans during the time of transatlantic slavery, many migrant agricultural workers, persons trafficked or kept confined for the purposes of sex work, and nonhuman animals "employed" in a variety of industries. Excluded, whether de jure (in law) or de facto (in reality), from full citizen status, the less than fully human subject haunts the margins of the global economic system as one whose labors enable the lifestyles of others and whose necessities of life are often framed as a drain on the "truly deserving" productive citizenry.

Finally, *legal* or *juridical* inclusion, or the protection of selected forms of life under the law, is a vital axis of categorizing living beings. In all modern states, even those with relatively progressive policies, regulations, and laws concerning noncitizens' "welfare," nonhumans possess much less protection from intentionally inflicted harm and death than do human beings. In most cases, the dominant framework of legal rights relating to nonhuman animals is one of *property*, with the focus of concern the financial consequences to the owner of the animal(s) in question or, occasionally, the potential loss to the broader human community of a sustained supply of resources (for example, wild fish populations) that might endanger economic stability.

Not only are those formally classed as nonhumans affected by this lack of legislative protection, however. Humans without state-issued documentation, belonging to particular ethnic groups, or possessing specific sets of physical or behavioral characteristics deemed "inferior" may, within a given politico-legal regime, be intentionally and systematically excluded from its aegis, often using the denial of "personhood" status.[32] By locating "animality" *within* some categories of *Homo sapiens*, Giorgio Agamben has argued, the modern world produces "animalized humans" who reside outside of the realm of protection of the law, as perpetually vulnerable "bare life"—a position akin to that of nonhuman animals.[33]

As partial and incomplete as the preceding list may be, it should be sufficient to give us a relatively clear idea of what is at stake in being deemed "human" or "animal," and why the animalization of the members of particular categories or collectivities has traditionally been of such concern in equity and human rights work. To be displaced from the status of full humanity, and, particularly, to be rendered as "animal," is, in the context of a deeply anthropocentric system, to be marginalized in the most fundamental of ways.

Furthermore, dehumanization as a rhetorical device and, hence, as a focal point of critique has a significant history embedded within it. Much of the propaganda associated with major historical oppressions and atrocities has included an explicit equation of particular human groups with nonhuman animals. Few persons raised within a North American or European cultural milieu would be at a loss to identify human groups or communities historically associated, through discriminatory rhetoric and representation, with species such as apes, dogs, or rats. Given these histories, the animalized caricaturization of even specific individuals, such as politicians or other public figures, who are also members of marginalized groups is usually identified by rights advocates as highly problematic.[34]

Here, Sara Ahmed's notion of the linguistic sign as a "sticky" system, one that accumulates both meaning and emotion through repeated associations,[35] may help us understand the ways in which condemnation of dehumanization as a tool of oppression has acquired not only *cognitive* meaning but also affective or "*felt*" value, and has become a repository for memories, experiences, and identities. These historical associations thus give the notion of dehumanization additional weight and depth, as it allows people to tie their own lived experiences of discrimination to well-recognized and widely condemned acts and events. The power of this idea to concisely convey the consequences of systematic prejudice and discrimination should not be dismissed lightly.

And yet, from the perspective of those who seek to expand intersectional equity frameworks to include nonhuman animals, the selection of "dehumanization" as the central point of critique remains problematic. While many of those who use the concept may not intend for their response to bleed foundational assumptions into spheres beyond human rights, this is difficult to avoid, given the literal, metaphorical, and affective suggestions of a human-nonhuman hierarchy implicit in "dehumanization."

Further—and potentially of great relevance even to those whose advocacy priorities do not extend to nonhuman beings—such usage may also contribute to the perpetuation of concrete relations of domination within and among human communities, as will be explored below. For such reasons, the concept and the ways in which it is deployed in the context of critique demands reevaluation.

In attending more closely to the issue of dehumanization as an analytical concept, I have chosen to focus on one particular form of bias, fat phobia, and its critique. Indeed, the intersections between anthropocentrism and anti-fat bias in general have been significantly undertheorized thus far, leaving the area ripe for exploration.

In both scholarly and advocacy work that is oriented toward countering size-based prejudice and discrimination, "dehumanization" is a common critique issued against representations of fat people in a variety of discourses and imagery. The application of this idea, I argue, stems from an understanding that such representations (especially when considered collectively) tend to situate fat people as "the excluded" along many, if not all, of the major axes of the human/nonhuman. Further, a "felt identification" on the part of those targeted by biased assumptions, forthright insults, or subtle "microaggressions"[36] with at least some of the affective associations of "dehumanization" as already established in other antioppressive movements (antiracism, feminism, disability advocacy, and so forth) also likely contributes to a willingness by many fat rights supporters to embrace the use of this established tactic of critique. While the marginalization faced by people of size may lack the dramatic "defining events" that mark the histories of some other forms of discrimination, the pervasive bias faced by many fat individuals in employment, education, health care, and other life spheres has generated a feeling of affinity among many proponents of size acceptance with the daily struggles faced by members of other oppressed communities.[37]

Indeed, in examining the sort of images and textual representations of fatness and fat subjects circulating in the public sphere and brought forth for critique by scholars and activists, one can readily see many of these same elements of exclusion at play. Media images often present fat people in ways that minimize or erase agency and subjectivity. Perhaps the clearest example of this phenomenon is the practice of news media using what fat activists often sardonically refer to as "headless fatties" photographs: images that capture fat individuals involved in some unremarkable but often stereotypical activity (eating is common, as is sitting in a relaxed pose), with the frame situated so as to exclude the person's face and, often, entire head.[38] The choice to use such representations does reveal an awareness by media outlets, ever fearful of lawsuits and compensatory payouts, of the expected opposition of the subjects of these photographs to the pairing of their bodies with negative commentary on fatness. But even more significant is the wealth of implicit meaning conveyed through the repetition of such images, in which fat individuals are symbolically decapitated, depersonalized, and silenced.

Medical literature and news reporting also often use objectifying rhetoric. Medical terminology itself may be inherently problematic; just as queer-positive, disability rights, and "mad pride" movements have fought against the use of categories and labels deemed stigmatizing ("invert," "invalid," "insane"), so too have size acceptance activists argued for the replacement of the language of medicalization ("overweight," "obese") with self-chosen identifiers ("fat," "persons of size"). Most revealing is the frequent use, in both medical sources and health-related media stories, of "person-absent" language—such as "*the* overweight" and "*the* obese"—which subsumes the individuality of fat persons into a generic, pathologized collective, where the act of "making meaning" of fatness is appropriated by professionals, and those meanings are then inscribed on fat bodies through medical discourses and practices. Such usage speaks to a vision of health-oriented communities as ones in which fatness is regarded as a signifier of exclusion from full and "proper" subjectivity, and as a marker of bodies to be studied and acted upon as the "raw materials" for the interests of nonfat "expert" subjects.

Following the lines of thought established by the pervasive nature-culture split, such representations tend to represent fat persons as excessively bound to physicality and distanced from the Enlightenment ideal of the "rational" intellect that has long held pride of place in modernity's conception of the human. Even in secular contexts, the philosophical and religio-ethical ideals of the restrained and disciplined subject are often deployed to cast the fat body as a supposed "confessor" of uncontrolled indulgence in "animalistic" desires.[39] The bodies of thin, "normal" subjects—especially if also white, male, heterosexual, and cisgender—tend to disappear from notice, while fat bodies are regarded as bearing stigmata of an orientation not toward the mind but in the direction of the "baser" drives for food and for rest. These are the very elements of the human that are considered points of (undesirable) connection with the nonhuman animal/natural realm, signs of "the animal (yet) within."

The fat person further tends to be represented as one who fails to meet the duties of the neoliberal responsibilized citizen. With the fat body discursively constituted through a blend of medical and other cultural discourses as a "high-maintenance" but nonproductive body, fat subjects become rendered as social and biopolitical "problems."[40] The alleged "excessive" fatness of the North American population has been blamed for problems ranging from a lack of military readiness,[41] to transportation safety problems,[42] to national economic decline.[43] Particularly where the United States is concerned, cultural associations of the nation with "fast-food"-style eating establishments and conveniences like widespread vehicle ownership have been combined with efforts to measure and tabulate population characteristics, bringing the idea of fatness as a defining, if disliked, national characteristic to the fore. So too has this prompted concerted efforts to remedy this supposed collective failing and restore the nation's Protestant-tinged image of self-reliant and disciplined productivity.[44] Within such a worldview, fat persons, individually and collectively, are constituted as a burden on, and potential endangerment to, the well-being and prosperity of the society and the nation-state.

Paradoxically, while the fatness of the population generates much moral consternation and attempts at systemic intervention—a phenomenon that, in fat activist circles, has prompted the popularization of the neologism "obesity epipanic"—concern for the well-being of individual fat persons often suffers the opposite fate. As, at best, a marginalized citizen within the body politic, the fat individual may at times be rendered as outside the mandate for equal protection by the law, in areas such as access to transportation,[45] medical treatment,[46] or parental rights.[47] In rare cases, fatness may even be used to justify subjecting particular individuals to the characteristic fate of Agamben's Homo sacer: the ability to be killed without that act being classed as "murder." (Such was the outcome, for example, of a 2010 British legal case in which a doctor was let off with only a £5,000 fine for causing the death of a fat woman in a vehicular accident, with the rationale: "If the person had been of average fitness they might have survived the injuries caused by the collision.")[48] More often, however, the "permitted" killing of the fat body may merely be carried out as a symbolic annihilation (as, for instance, in the advertisements of a Brazilian dairy products company, in which fat bodies become converted into shooting gallery-style targets, accompanied by the tagline, "Adeus gordura": "Goodbye, fat").[49]

In addition to the often covert references to this network of interconnected ideas that endorse lesser social, cultural, moral, and political statuses for fat human beings, there are also those representations that more overtly make the equation between fatness and animality. Notable for its clarity of intent is an ad campaign for a Romanian weight loss spa that presents a trio of representations of thin, toned human figures "evolving" out of animal bodies—a cow, a pig, and a whale.[50] Such images provide a vivid confirmation of the underlying logic that continually works to reproduce the marginalization of those subjects who inhabit fat bodies.

Perhaps most startling, however, is encountering representations of this sort produced and promoted not by diet food producers or weight loss organizations, but by animal rights groups. Among the most (in)famous, a large billboard in Jacksonville, Florida, erected by People for the Ethical Treatment of Animals (PETA), depicts an illustration of a fat woman in a red-and-white polka-dot bikini, facing away from the viewer as she gazes upon the sun-dappled ocean in front of her. This scene, however, is not intended to depict a satisfied woman enjoying a pleasant day at the beach—for the text accompanying the image reads "Save the Whales—Lose the Blubber: Go Vegetarian."[51] Leaving aside the problematic assumption that fat bodies are necessarily meat-eating bodies, one might expect that an animal rights organization would be well situated to understand what is at stake in attempting to stigmatize certain human beings by animalizing them. A charitable conclusion would be that the existence of advertisements of this sort suggests, at the least, a lack of conscious awareness of the underlying logics of intersecting varieties of bias-driven degradation and marginalization.

Like other forms of bias—though their consequences may differ quite radically in kind and, especially, in severity—both the stigmatization of fat persons and the exploitation of nonhuman animals ultimately rest upon the belief that some lives are inherently "lacking" and, therefore, legitimately devalued along social, cultural, political, and other axes. But how, then, might this recognition be rendered into meaningful, transformative practice by those engaged in critical, intersectional equity-oriented work? A few tentative suggestions may be in order.

For fat acceptance activists, scholars, and allies, it is imperative to question the full implications of using dehumanization as a cardinal point of critique and to ask what broader systems of power are actually being perpetuated in so doing. Those who seek to foster the emergence of a world free from fat phobia might do well to start a conversation around alternative ways of answering back to discriminatory rhetoric that do not depend on the deployment of "dehumanization." Might we, as persons committed to ensuring individuals of all sizes and of all species have the opportunity to experience rich and meaningful lives, instead call upon language that speaks with more specificity to the actions being performed on and toward subjects when they are "dehumanized"? Is it possible to expand and/or reframe other established concepts and terminology—like "objectification" or "thingification"—to encompass much of the territory that we presently try to capture with the label of

"dehumanization," building upon the fact that those terms address discriminatory rhetoric or images without identifying humanity-versus-animality as the
fundamental point of contention? In cases where actual animalized representations of fat persons or other marginalized human subjects are at issue, explicitly addressing the underlying forms of exclusion intended (e.g., impaired
intellect, lack of self-control, substandard cleanliness), rather than the
imputed nonhuman status per se, is one possibility for framing an antiexcep-
tionalist critique.

Perhaps there might even be value in crafting *new* terms in a quest to holis-
tically capture the commonalities of various oppressions without inadvertently
marginalizing nonhuman animals. Granted, novel terminology would lack the
historical force that has fused itself to "dehumanization." But, as Ahmed's
work suggests, new words can also become "sticky" and, like snowballs, gather
meaning, affect, and power the more we roll them around in our discourses
and our critiques.

Further, in creating alternative counterdiscourses to existing oppressive or
marginalizing ones, it is important to carefully think through their full consequences. For example, it is not uncommon for size acceptance activists to
frame their opposition to the surveillance and stigmatization of fat people's
consumption practices by decisively rejecting any moralization of dietary
choices.[52] While the motives for this are quite understandable, blanket
declarations of food as out of bounds for ethical or political debate contribute
to erasing the suffering, exploitation, and death—of humans as well as of
nonhumans—that are involved in some forms of food production. In a
capitalist economy, it is difficult to ignore the role of consumer choices in perpetuating such practices; personal dietary choices are inherently embedded
with issues of power and privilege. An approach that closes down possibilities
for dialogue and critique on these matters will clearly pose an obstacle to
constructive discussion between those invested in body diversity acceptance
and those committed to advocacy on behalf of nonhuman animals.

Reciprocally, for those who profess a primary commitment to animal rights,
it should be evident that endorsing discourses that act to stigmatize, pathologize, or otherwise marginalize certain types of human subjects is not ultimately
in the interests of nonhuman animals. Because different types of living beings
partake, to varying degrees, in a shared body of assumptions concerning the
characteristics that qualify or disqualify an individual from full standing as a
subject and agent, perpetuating biases along these axes only reinforces the
very criteria of exclusion themselves. Working to find approaches to airing
concerns around the status and treatment of nonhumans, while still acknowledging and addressing the ways that fat-phobic policing of bodies and habits
creates ongoing hardships for fat people (and others), is a necessity for
effective and compassionate interspecies advocacy. Indeed, as Haraway has

argued, there is merit in shifting the core of the discussion from one of "rights" to one of "ethical relating"[53]—specifically of working to foster, in feminist philosopher Chris Cuomo's words, an "ethic of flourishing"[54]—that respects differences and calls us to an "ongoing alertness to otherness-in-relation."[55] As long as bodily differences are employed as justifications for restricting opportunities for participation in social, cultural, political, and other life spheres, neither the animal nor the "animalized" will escape the relentless undertow of the logics of human exceptionalism.

In practical terms, a commitment to intersectional resistance also entails an obligation to think critically about the animal advocacy projects and organizations one opts to support. Ethical imperatives in equity work are inescapable. When deciding to engage in collective efforts, one is often confronted with the need to make conscientious choices about whether or not to endorse a particular group, but also with the question of whether to commit to working *within* problematic activist communities with the goal of reforming them. Participation within broader networks of advocacy carries with it the possibility of greater results—but also the responsibility to attend to the more significant ancillary effects and to take measures to shape these in positive and productive ways. For example, it is particularly important that critical animal scholarship and animal rights activism interrogate the specific ways in which appeals to discourses of "health promotion" are employed to advocate for a lifestyle that benefits animals. From the perspective of the size acceptance movement, there is a pressing need to self-consciously decouple discourses of health and wellness—endorsed by many animal rights groups, and the keystone of ones such as the Physicians Committee for Responsible Medicine—from weight loss promotion. This is not only because it appears to be untrue that most people who turn to a plant-based diet will experience substantial permanent weight changes,[56] but because devaluing and stigmatizing fat bodies also contributes indirectly to entrapping nonhuman animals within these shared exclusionary logics. No less significantly, promoting weight-oriented health claims contributes to making animal rights communities chilly, or even hostile, climates for fat participants, reducing the commitment and potential contributions of those whose bodies fail to conform to contemporary cultural ideals—as well as, consequently, perpetuating the pejorative image of "herbivores" as of a uniform physical type.

While there is much room for improvement in crafting progressive spaces that take into account intersectionality around issues of animal rights and size acceptance, there are, nevertheless, already a few heartening developments to be found. Some individuals who have allegiances to both fat-positive values and proanimal causes are seeking new and creative ways of addressing this matrix of interrelated oppressions, resisting antifat bias and the erasure of fat subjectivity without reinscribing the devaluation of the animal. Notable among these is a U.S.-based artist, who goes by only her first name, Christie; she has created and disseminated online a clever visual statement by way of response to PETA's "Save the Whales" billboard. Posing her own bikini-clad fat body in front of a picturesque shoreline in mimicry of the PETA image, she inscribes the image with a different sort of textual message: "I am a vegetarian but I am still a 'whale.' "[57] In opting not to refute the animalistic characterization of the original advertisement but, rather, to embrace it in a defiant fashion and inscribe it with a countermessage to that of the original, the overall effect is a subversion of sorts, which takes aim at the underlying fat-phobic dimension of the original representation. Looking at this parodic image, the viewer is challenged to simultaneously rethink dominant cultural messages about the devaluation of animality and the nature of fatness. Efforts like this, I would argue, have a valuable role to play in bridging the divide between activist communities. If there is one key conviction that needs to be brought to the table in intersectional equity work, it is that *everyone* is inextricably bound within a collective struggle for greater freedom and new possibilities of living.

NOTES

1. Kimberlé Crenshaw, "Demarginalizing the Intersection of Sex and Race: A Black Feminist Critique of Antidiscrimination Doctrine, Feminist Theory and Antiracist Politics," *University of Chicago Legal Forum* (1989): 139.

2. See Kathy Davis, "Intersectionality as Buzzword: A Sociology of Science Perspective on What Makes a Feminist Theory Successful," *Feminist Theory* 9, no. 1 (2008): 67–85.

3. Jennifer C. Nash, "Re-thinking Intersectionality," *Feminist Review* 89 (2008): 3.

4. Arlene Stein, "Make Room for Daddy: Anxious Masculinity and Emergent Homophobias in Neopatriarchal Politics," *Gender and Society* 19, no. 5 (2005): 601–20.

5. Ingunn Moser, "Sociotechnical Practices and Difference: On the Interferences between Disability, Gender, and Class," *Science, Technology, & Human Values* 31, no. 5 (2006): 537–64.

6. See Colleen Mack-Canty, "Third-Wave Feminism and the Need to Reweave the Nature/Culture Duality," *NWSA Journal* 16, no. 3 (2004): 154–79.

7. For example, see the special issue of *Journal for Critical Animal Studies* on "Women of Color in Critical Animal Studies," guest editors Anastasia Yarbrough and Susan Thomas, vol. 8, no. 3 (2010).

8. Daniel Salomon, "From Marginal Cases to Linked Oppressions: Reframing the Conflict between the Autistic Pride and Animal Rights Movements," *Journal for Critical Animal Studies* 8, nos. 1/2 (2010): 47–72.

9. See Donna Haraway, *The Companion Species Manifesto* (Chicago: Prickly Paradigm, 2003), and *When Species Meet* (Minneapolis: University of Minnesota Press, 2007).

10. Jacques-Philippe Leyens has coined the term "infrahumanization" to refer to the process of attributing differential degrees of "humanness" to various human groups (see Jacques-Phillippe Leyens, "Retrospective and Prospective Thoughts about Infrahumanization," *Group Processes and Intergroup Relations* 12, no. 6 (2009): 807–17). The term itself, while embraced by some researchers of social behavior, nevertheless shares many of the problematic aspects of "dehumanization," given its suggestion of a human-nonhuman hierarchy.

11. The latter is often also referred to as size acceptance, body diversity acceptance, fat rights, or fat liberation. Though each of these terms has certain unique connotations, for the purposes of this chapter they are used more or less interchangeably.

12. For an analysis of various perspectives on categories in intersectional scholarship, see Leslie McCall, "The Complexity of Intersectionality," *Journal of Women in Culture and Society* 30, no. 3 (2005): 1771–1800.

13. See, for example, Daniel Elstein, "Species as a Social Construction: Is Species Morally Relevant?," *Journal for Critical Animal Studies* 1, no. 1 (2003): n.p.; Johanna Tito, "On Animal Immortality: An Argument for the Possibility of Animal Immortality in Light of the History of Philosophy," in *Animal Subjects*, ed. J. Castricano (Waterloo, Ontario: WLU Press, 2008), 285–300; Hasana Sharp, "Animal Affects: Spinoza and the Frontiers of the Human," *Journal for Critical Animal Studies* 9, nos. 1/2 (2011): 48–68.

14. Notable examples include Harriet Ritvo, *The Animal Estate: The English and Other Creatures in the Victorian Age* (Cambridge, MA: Harvard University Press, 1987), and *Noble Cows and Hybrid Zebras: Essays on Animals and History* (Charlottesville: University of Virginia Press, 2010); also, Graham D. Burnett, *Trying Leviathan: The Nineteenth-Century New York Court Case That Put the Whale on Trial and Challenged the Order of Nature* (Princeton, NJ: Princeton University Press, 2007).

15. Most significant, perhaps, are Giorgio Agamben, *The Open: Man and Animal* (Palo Alto, CA: Stanford University Press, 2004), and Jacques Derrida, *The Animal That Therefore I Am* (New York: Fordham University Press, 2008).

16. Kay Anderson's monograph *Race and the Crisis of Humanism* (London: Routledge, 2007) is pioneering in the regard. See also Anderson's article "Culture and Nature at the Adelaide Zoo: At the Frontiers of 'Human' Geography," *Transactions, Institute of British Geographers* 20, no. 3 (1995): 275–94.

17. Besides Haraway's work, see also the interdisciplinary *Society and Animals* journal (Brill, 1993–present), and the "Multispecies Ethnography" special issue of *Cultural Anthropology* 25, no. 4 (2010).

18. For example, see "Culture" in *Cultural Theory: The Key Concepts*, ed. Andrew Edgar and Peter Sedgwick (London: Routledge, 2002), 101–3.

19. George F. MacDonald, "What Is Culture?," *Journal of Museum Education* 16, no. 1 (1991): 9–12.

20. See Gregory Radick, *The Simian Tongue: The Long Debate about Animal Language* (Chicago: University of Chicago Press, 2008).

21. Bryan S. Turner, "Recent Developments in the Theory of the Body," in *The Body: Social Process and Cultural Theory*, ed. M. Featherstone, M. Hepworth, and B. Turner (London: Sage, 1991), 17.

22. See Chris Shilling, *The Body and Social Theory* (London: Sage, 2003), esp. chap. 3, "The Naturalistic Body," 37–61.

23. For a lucid overview of these varying worldviews and ethics, see David Kinsley, *Ecology and Religion: Ecological Spirituality in Cross-Cultural Perspective* (Englewood Cliffs, NJ: Prentice Hall, 1995).

24. H. Paul Santmire, *The Travail of Nature: The Ambiguous Ecological Promise of Christian Theology* (Philadelphia: Fortress Press, 1985).

25. Kinsley, *Ecology and Religion*, chap. 8: "Christianity as Ecologically Harmful," 103–14.

26. For examples from major thinkers in Western history, see Gary Steiner, *Anthropocentrism and Its Discontents: The Moral Status of Animals in the History of Western Philosophy* (Pittsburgh, PA: University of Pittsburgh Press, 2005).

27. A foundational text in this regard is Peter Singer's *Animal Liberation* (New York: Avon, 1975).

28. Kelly Oliver, *Animal Lessons: How They Teach Us to Be Human* (New York: Columbia University Press, 2009).

29. Margaret R. Somers and Christopher N. J. Roberts, "Toward a New Sociology of Rights: A Genealogy of 'Buried Bodies' of Citizenship and Human Rights," *Annual Review of Law and Social Science* 4 (December 2008): 385–425.

30. See Tina Besley and Michael A. Peters, *Subjectivity and Truth: Foucault, Education, and the Culture of Self* (New York: Peter Lang, 2007).

31. See Bob Torres, *Making a Killing: The Political Economy of Animal Rights* (Oakland, WV: AK Press, 2007).

32. For an example of an exceptionalist perspective on "personhood" (including some attention to its role in delineating humans from other animals) see Heikki Ikäheimo, "A Vital Human Need: Recognition as Inclusion in Personhood," *European Journal of Political Theory* 8, no. 1 (2009): 31–45.

33. See Agamben, *The Open*.

34. For an example of controversy surrounding animal imagery and racialized signification, see Oliver Burkeman, "New York Post in Racism Row over Chimpanzee Cartoon," *Guardian*, February 18, 2009, http://www.guardian.co.uk/world/2009/feb/18/new-york-post-cartoon-race.

35. Sara Ahmed, *The Cultural Politics of Emotion* (New York: Routledge, 2004), 90–92.

36. The term "microaggression," now commonplace in the studies of systematic bias, refers to "minor" acts or expressions of prejudicial thought or feeling, sometimes unconscious/unintentional, encountered by members of stigmatized groups within the ordinary spheres of daily life. See Chester M. Pierce et al., "An Experiment in Racism: TV Commercials," *Education and Urban Society* 10, no. 1 (1977): 61– 87.

37. Marilyn Wann, "Fat Studies: An Invitation to Revolution," in *The Fat Studies Reader*, ed. Esther Rothblum and Sondra Solovay (New York: New York University Press, 2009), ix–xxv.

38. For an example of size acceptance advocates' perspectives on this phenomenon, see Kate Harding's piece, and the ensuing discussion in the comments: "Open Thread: Headless Fatties," *Shapely Prose* (blog), February 6, 2009, http://kateharding.net/2009/02/06/open-thread-headless-fatties/.

39. See Sander L. Gilman, *Fat: A Cultural History of Obesity* (Cambridge: Polity, 2008), especially chap. 3, "The Stigma of Obesity," 78–100.

40. See Jan Wright and Valerie Harwood, eds., *Biopolitics and the "Obesity Epidemic": Governing Bodies* (London: Taylor & Francis, 2008).

41. John Cawley and Johanna Catherine Maclean, "Unfit for Service: The Implications of Rising Obesity for U.S. Military Recruitment," NBER Working Paper No. 16408, September 2010, http://www.nber.org/papers/w16408.pdf.

42. Larry Copeland, "Overweight Americans Throwing Off Safety of City Buses," *USA Today*, April 31, 2011, http://www.usatoday.com/yourlife/fitness/2011-03-21-busweight21_ST_N.htm. Also: "Deadly Decision: Obese Drivers Are Far Less Likely to Buckle Up," *University at Buffalo/Newswise*, April 27, 2012, http://www.newswise.com/articles/deadly-decision-obese-drivers-are-far-less-likely-to-buckle-up.

43. Andre Picard, "Obesity Costs Economy Up to $7-Billion a Year," *Globe & Mail*, June 20, 2011, http://www.theglobeandmail.com/life/health/new-health/conditions/obesity/obesity-costs-economy-up-to-7-billion-a-year/article2068087/. Also, see Michelle Obama's comments on the alleged economic impact of childhood obesity in the United States: "Remarks by the First Lady at National League of Cities Conference," The White House, March 15, 2011, http://www.whitehouse.gov/the-press-office/2011/03/15/remarks-first-lady-national-league-cities-conference.

44. J. Eric Oliver, *Fat Politics: The Real Story behind America's Obesity Epidemic* (New York: Oxford University Press, 2006), esp. chap.7, "Sloth, Capitalism, and the Paradox of Freedom," 143–58.

45. Joyce L. Huff, "Access to the Sky: Airplane Seats and Fat Bodies as Contested Spaces," in Rothblum and Solovay, *The Fat Studies Reader*.

46. For instance, in the United States, hospital policies routinely prohibit life-saving organ transplants to persons with a body mass index exceeding a given level, even in the absence of other health-related limitations. Also, for examples of views regarding medical care and fatness in the UK, see Denis Campbell, "Doctors Back Denial of Treatment for Smokers and the Obese," *Guardian*, April 29, 2012, http://www.guardian.co.uk/society/2012/apr/28/doctors-treatment-denial-smokers-obese.

47. See, for example, Martin Beckford, "Take Obese Children into Care, Says Health Expert," *Telegraph*, October 3, 2008, http://www.telegraph.co.uk/health/3130908/Take-obese-children-into-care-says-health-expert.html. Also, regarding China's exclusion of fat persons from international adoptions, see Jim Yardley, "China Tightens Adoption Rules, U.S. Agencies Say," *New York Times*, December 19, 2006, http://www.nytimes.com/2006/12/19/world/asia/19cnd-adopt.html?_r=1.

48. "Fine for Doctor Who Killed an Obese Woman," STV News [Scotland], November 16, 2010, http://news.stv.tv/tayside/209483-fine-for-doctor-who-killed-an-obese-woman/.

49. "Fat Criminals ARE Easier to Shoot," *Copyranter* (blog), March 15, 2010, http://copyranter.blogspot.ca/2010/03/fat-criminals-are-easier-to-shoot.html.

50. "Next Stop on the Worldwide Sexist Ad Tour: Romania," *Copyranter* (blog), August 5, 2008, http://copyranter.blogspot.ca/2008/08/next-stop-on-worldwide-sexist-ad-tour.html.

51. Katherine Goldstein, "PETA's New 'Save the Whales' Billboard Takes Aim at Fat Women," *Huffington Post*, September 26, 2009, http://www.huffingtonpost.com/2009/08/26/petas-new-save-the-whales_n_261134.html.

52. See, for example, fat acceptance advocate Marianne Kirby's piece, "Food for Thought; If All Food Choices Are Valid, That Means ALL Food Choices," *The Rotund* (blog), April 22, 2011, http://www.therotund.com/?p=1143.

53. Haraway, *The Companion Species Manifesto*, 50.

54. Chris Cuomo, *Feminism and Ecological Communities: An Ethic of Flourishing* (New York: Routledge, 2002); referenced in Haraway, *The Companion Species Manifesto*, 54.

55. Haraway, *The Companion Species Manifesto*, 50.

56. Data on the "success rates" of vegetarian/vegan diets for long-term weight loss are scanty at best; however, studies of a wide variety of weight loss methods (inclusive of diets that are primarily plant based) have found little data to support the contention that *any* particular form of dietary modification is effective, on the whole, for producing significant and sustained weight loss (see Glenn Gaesser, "Is 'Permanent Weight Loss' an Oxymoron?," in Rothblum and Solovay, *The Fat Studies Reader*, 37–41). Weight-related claims about vegetarian diets often rely on research showing a modest average weight differential between vegetarians and nonvegetarians, but these data frequently ignore potential confounding factors, such as research participants' ethnic origins, socioeconomic status, and perceived acceptance within vegetarian/vegan communities.

57. Christie, "PETA's Anti-fat 'Whale' Campaign," *Inside the Mind of a Creepy Dollmaker* (blog), August 24, 2009, http://bastet2329.blogspot.com/2009/08/petas-anti-fat-whale-campaign.html

18

5F: On Being Different and Loving It!

Nadav (Nadiva) Antebi

I weigh 280 pounds. I am fat. I do not care about gender roles. I am fem. I am more attracted to men. I am a fag. I love my beautiful self and my sexy body. I am fabulous. I never apologize for who I am and what I am. I am fierce. I am 5F.

ON BEING MENTALLY AND PHYSICALLY FAT

I have always been different and I love it! But being different has its price. Since the age of five, I have been considered by others to be a fat kid, which already then made me different from the other kids. When you are a kid, however, being fat can be cute and endearing. So I was different, but I was cute. Unfortunately, that did not last for too long, and in elementary school things started to change. I cannot say that I was bullied and harassed on a daily basis, nor can I say that I was popular and loved by my schoolmates. The only thing I am certain of is that I was different. More importantly, I felt different. This feeling of otherness was translated back then to discomfort and even frustration that in turn resulted in bullying—where I was the bully and not the victim. I was mean, aggressive, and verbally violent toward my classmates and my teachers. Incidents of bullying are very vague in my memory from elementary school, but I remember I was constantly asked, "How can you be that mean to others?" Thinking back, I believe it was a destructive tactic to ask for a "place at the table" among my peers. It was also a somewhat creative technique to justify to myself why I was considered to be so different from others. My aggression and verbal violence served as a rationalization system that provided the very simple explanation as to why I was different and got treated differently. If you are mean and aggressive toward others, even if only with hurtful words, you are most likely to become an outcast (i.e., different). This violence and sense of otherness led to a spiral of negative consequences, some of which were getting terrible grades in all of my classes, feeling even more lonely than usual, and making my parents come to school at least once a week to discuss my situation and performance at school. This vicious cycle had to be broken somehow, and one way to do that was by addressing my sense of otherness.

When I was in the fourth grade I weighed 135 pounds. I was fat, a very bad student, a bully, and hated by all. Back then, I believed that my fat was the easiest to alter, thinking that having a thinner figure would make me feel less different and that I was like my classmates who were mostly slimmer than me. I joined Weight Watchers, and over the course of six months I lost 18 pounds. It was not a success story. It took me only five months to gain those 18 pounds back, with an additional 10 pounds. I was still very different, even more than before. But that is not the whole story. During the end of my fourth-grade year, my parents decided to get a divorce. I remember being in a state of shock when my father told me that he had a girlfriend and that he was moving in with her as soon as possible. Up to that moment, I was positive that my parents were the most loving couple in the world. Clearly, that was not the case. I felt betrayed by my father, and I became angry at the world. I was verbally violent toward my peers and treated food (mostly snacks and candy) as my comfort.

It was not until I witnessed my two older brothers dealing with my parents' divorce that I realized that something had to be done differently. I felt that not speaking with my father as an act of resentment for abandoning us was somewhat immature. I decided to act in what I thought was a more mature way. I asked to see a child psychologist. The therapy lasted for about a year and was successful as it had a major positive impact on my development. I can certainly say that it changed my life. I became calmer, I was not aggressive or verbally violent anymore, and I was finally getting good grades in all of my classes, including physical education, despite the fact that I did not enjoy it.

Along with the mental healing process, my mom and I thought that it would be a good idea to go on another diet. We had the chance to meet a nutrition expert who was visiting Israel (where I was born and lived until the age of 26) from the United States. We both placed our hopes in her knowledge and experience and followed everything she asked us to do. After a comprehensive battery of blood and allergy tests, I was told that I was lactose-intolerant. For a 12-year-old kid with a big love for ice cream, pizza, and chocolate, it meant eliminating more than 70 percent of my daily diet. I still suspect that this "lactose-intolerance" diagnosis was a complete lie meant to make me refrain from eating foods high in fat, sugar, and carbs. Along with a controlled low-fat and low-carb diet, I managed to lose 35 pounds. In my head, I was still very fat.

I started middle school thinner than I had ever been, which made me feel less different compared to my classmates. This fresh start brought along a social life that I did not really have during elementary school. I became more popular and made more friends. Slowly, I was so consumed by my social life and hanging out with my new friends that I did not bother to study or do my homework. My oldest brother, to whom I am grateful to this day, decided to take action. In the beginning of my second semester of seventh grade, my brother made sure I completed all the homework assignments, added dictations in English, and wrote tests to ensure my progress in school. My brother's surveillance turned me into a straight A student. I completed the seventh grade with excellent final grades in all of my classes. Then, it was the eighth grade. I was mainly concentrating on my classes, hanging out with friends from time to time, and gaining weight. By the end of the eighth grade, my grades were still excellent and I was fat again.

Ninth grade started and along with it, my eating disorder. Once and for all, I decided to exterminate my sense of fatness. I wanted to get rid of all my body fat and, most importantly, eradicate my self-perception as a fat individual. I just could not handle being different anymore and not feeling like I belonged. I followed the "simple" formula: less food = fewer calories = weight loss. I ate one big bowl of salad a day and nothing else. I also started exercising out of my own will for the first time in my life and took at least one spinning or kickboxing class a day. Obviously, as a result, I lost a significant amount of weight. Presumably, everything was working in my favor. I was slim, I had friends, I was a great student, and I felt better overall. However, in my mind I was still very fat and wanted to lose even more weight. I then went to a nutritionist so she could advise me and suggest other successful weight loss techniques. She weighed me and after I told her that I came in for weight loss purposes, she started asking me weird questions, like if I eat frozen foods straight from the freezer without cooking or heating them up first. I responded that this was absolutely not the case. A few years later, I realized that she was screening me for having some sort of an eating disorder. She was shocked to discover that I saw myself as a fat person. Back then, I did not quite understand what she was thinking and why she was so shocked. I genuinely did not see myself as thin, slim, or in any way not fat. In my own perception, I was fat. Five years after my meeting with the nutritionist, I remember looking at older photos of mine and realizing how thin I actually was back then. She sat me down for a talk and told me that she hates to be the bearer of bad news but that I have an eating disorder. After I completely rejected everything she said, and especially my "newly discovered clinical diagnosis," she insisted that I was absolutely thin and within the right weight-height ratio, and that the last thing I should worry about is losing weight. I, on the other hand, was not at all convinced. I continued with my not-healthy-at-all diet until mid-August of that year, a terribly hot and humid time of the year in Tel-Aviv, when I found myself constantly exhausted every day. Clearly, it was because I did not consume enough calories to provide me with sufficient energy to last for a whole day. I became lethargic, moody, and less social than before. Easily enough, I started eating again. I slowly gained more weight, but unlike past diets, this time I managed to maintain a "healthy" weight. In my own mind, on the other hand, I was becoming fatter, which meant that the incongruence between the self-perception of my body and weight, and my actual weight was dramatically distorted. Tenth grade had started and nothing was out of the ordinary. I remember that year as a very relaxed and somewhat uneventful one compared to my past school years. School was going well for me, I had a few close friends, and although I was certainly not perceived as fat by others, I still felt fat. Eleventh and 12th grades were quite similar to my experience in the 10th grade. A few pounds more or less throughout the years, but my stubborn self-perception as a fat person persisted regardless of my actual weight.

In Israel, after graduating from high school, both men and women are enlisted into a compulsory military service. Those were, by far, the worst three years of my life. I hated every minute of it. As someone who experienced stigmatization, rejection, and verbal violence (as both the aggressor and the victim), I absolutely resisted any form of aggression, violence, or domination. I was and still am a passionate pacifist, and the military was the last thing on my mind. I tried to get away with not serving, but it did not work for me. Unfortunately and unfairly, the Israeli Defense Forces does not discharge people from serving in the military for reasons of conscience or pacifism. I was practically forced into serving in the Israeli army for three years, and if that is not enough, I was stationed in an army base in the Gaza Strip, which was a central war zone back then. I had to carry a rifle on my back 24/7 and to place it under my pillow during my sleep. As they say in the military, "Your rifle is like your third arm"—you always have to carry it with you wherever you go. Although I was in the middle of a war zone, I did not serve as a combat soldier. I served as the coordination and liaison officer for the humanitarian aid (e.g., foods, drugs, and other basic supplies) entering into the Gaza Strip with the generous help of different humanitarian agencies such as UNRWA, the Red Cross, and Doctors Without Borders. One might think I at least got an officer position that is beneficial and in favor of the Palestinian people living in Gaza, but I just did not want and still do not want to have anything with the Israeli Defense Forces. I regret every moment I spent there. I felt depressed, down, and wanted it to be over with. Once again, I felt like a misfit that will never acclimate to the new forced "habitat."

Besides the friends I made, who were the best I ever had, one of whom is still very dear and close, my comfort was food. Every military base in Israel has a dining hall where soldiers, officers, and other staff congregate for breakfast, lunch, and dinner. Some of those dining halls are fancier than others. When you serve in an army base that due to its mission and distance from your home requires you to stay there and visit your home only once every other weekend, you are pampered with the best food an army base dining hall can offer. My few close friends as well as the delicious food served as my support system. My mental health was not at all perfect, to say the least. Consequently, in less than a year, I gained more than 60 pounds. I was the fattest I had ever been. I knew that something had to be done in order to change the miserable state I was in. After repeated begging to move to another base that would allow me to be closer to home, I was finally stationed in a military base in Tel-Aviv, a 10-minute walking distance from where I lived at the time. I had one more year of military service before being discharged. I decided to try and improve my mental and physical health and went on another diet. This time it was a very controlled one, accompanied by an uncontrolled amount of exercising. At the end of my last year in the army, I had lost 66 pounds and felt relieved and content. It was a very happy time in my life when I finally got discharged.

But still, not everything was getting better. This incongruence between my self-perception and actual weight persisted. Once again, I was thin but still thought of myself as a fat person. As a post-military service gift to myself, I flew to Baltimore, Maryland, to work as a dance instructor at a summer camp. The United States, for me, was a land of an overwhelming diversity of foods, most of which were delicious, yet high in calories, fat, and sugars. As part of the experience of living in the United States for three months, I did not want to miss any opportunity to try new and delicious foods, of any kind. I was stunned by the sizes of the supermarkets in Maryland, the serving sizes in restaurants and cafes, and the infinite (or so it seemed to me) variety of foods. I wanted to try it all. And so I did. Not surprisingly, it took me only three months to gain back the weight I had lost earlier that year. When I got back to Israel, I was fat again. From that moment on, there would be only more weight gain. I currently weigh 280 pounds.

For most of my life, I did not conform to gender roles. In fact, excluding specific periods during middle school and high school, trying to fit in, I never conformed to gender roles and found them irrelevant to me. Since I was a little kid, I loved to act and perform. My mom says that I gave my first performance when I was only three years old. She says I used to go into my dearest grandmother's closet and try on every single dress she had. It turns out from the pictures that I had a particular affinity for floral spring dresses. I never neglected my grandmother's impressive collection of shoes and, more specifically, the pumps. After choosing the best outfit for the event, I asked my entire family to find a seat before my performance had begun and directed them when to applaud during the show. I remembered I enjoyed every moment on the "stage."

Tracing back to kindergarten, during Purim (the Israeli "Halloween"), I remember all the boys dressed up as Spiderman and only I dressed up as Cinderella, simply because I found her prettier. Interestingly, I do not remember any negative comments from other kids. At the age of five, I gave my first show in "full drag." I lip synced to one of my favorite songs by my all-time favorite Israeli diva, Rita. Up to this day I am highly impressed by my drag skills as a little kid. My oldest brother also remembers coming back home from school and finding me with my mom's makeup smeared all over my face. I believe that the fact that feminine aesthetics were, in my eyes, more colorful, liberating, expressive, and overall fun is what drew my attention to them. One of the things I vividly remember and very much appreciate is that every member of my family was always enthusiastic and supportive about my gender nonconformity and passion for the performing arts during my childhood.

In elementary school, I experienced bullying because of my gender nonconformity. I was called names and harassed not too frequently but frequently enough to feel bad and embarrassed about it. Kids, like adults, conflate gender nonconformity with nonheterosexual orientation, so that if you do not conform to stereotypical gender roles and norms, you must be gay, queer, or a fag. These are only three of the comments my schoolmates used to make about my gender performance, the way I talked, or the way I moved. Being fat with a pear-shaped body has given my body an even more feminized look. Combined with being stigmatized for being fat, I learned that it was better if I try to conceal and hide any gender-nonconforming feature I had. I started playing soccer during recess even though I did not enjoy it. I tried to wear more conforming clothes but did not care for them at all. I tried to observe and monitor the gestures of the cool kids and imitate them. It did not really work for me. I think it would be fair to say that it did not take long until I decided to simply embrace my gender nonconformity while still trying to fit it, or at least not to stand out.

My mother worked and still works for the most renowned theater in Israel. Therefore, from very early on, I was familiar with the backstage and front stage of the theater and was enchanted by both. I knew I wanted to be part of it, and more as a performer, at the very front of the stage. At the age of seven, I asked my mom if she would sign me up for ballet classes since I wanted to become a ballet dancer. She politely suggested that I would be teased and ridiculed for wearing tight clothes as dancers typically do. I thought it was a good enough reason to abandon that idea. I then asked if I could become a theater actor. I got another negative response, this time based on the argument that it is challenging to be an actor and to make a decent living out of it. I had to put this dream aside as well. Thankfully, different events during elementary school allowed me to experiment with the performing arts. For every holiday event we had in school, I got the leading role, sometimes even a typically female role, and was received with raving applause. One of the events where I was, and am, particularly surprised at how well I was received was the bat mitzvah party for all the girls in my class, in which I performed in "full drag" to the song "Diva" by Dana International, the most famous trans* female singer in Israel.

Middle school and high school were my gray days, where I remember trying harder to fit in, though not overly so. Maybe that is why those days are vaguer in my memory. From what I can remember, I tried being myself; that is, I tried not to conceal any of my characteristics, but at the same time, not to stand out too much. I wanted to simply "pass," to use stigma-related terms. I did not want to be singled out because of my performance so I was trying to go under people's radar. That being said, it is important to emphasize that in my perception and feeling, I did not "cover" or completely alter the way I looked, moved, talked, or acted.

During my military service, and especially during my time spent in the Gaza Strip, I was extremely flamboyant (with the limitations of being a soldier). I remember being such a huge diva and overperforming every gesture and movement. I believed my exaggerated and over-the-top gender-nonconforming performance were my coping mechanisms to deal with the mental struggles I had to face during my military service. Shockingly or not, I do not remember even one incident of bashing, ridicule, or even teasing because of my gender nonconformity. In fact, my performance was my trademark and gave other people the impression that I was a brave and unique individual.

Ever since my military service, I celebrate my gender nonconformity and enjoy the range of opportunities and possibilities it opened for me. Not being bound to stereotypical gender roles and norms has allowed me to be a freer spirit than people who do care about these rules and work to abide by them. More importantly, my gender nonconformity has been and still is a real blessing as it enabled my open-minded and fluid perspective about what it means to be a social actor in our society.

The first time I told myself that I might be attracted to men was when I was 10 years old. I had to fill out an application in order to see a child psychologist after my parents got divorced in which I was asked what issues bothered me and why I want to meet with a therapist. One of the reasons I listed was that I thought I was attracted to boys. As the focus of the therapy sessions were mainly around my parents' divorce, we did not get enough chances to address that issue. I assume I was not mentally ready to explicitly discuss it with another person.

At the age of 14, I confronted my sexual orientation. I did not know much about what it meant to be nonheterosexual. I went on the Internet and started looking for every bit of information I could find about lesbian, gay, bisexual, transgender, and queer (LGBTQ) individuals. I was delighted to find enough information online to know that I am not the only one having the same emotions and thoughts. I also learned a lot of negative things about being LGBTQ: I learned that we smoke and abuse substance; we have conflicts with our friends and family; we are marginalized and stigmatized; we are bullied, teased, ridiculed, and discriminated against; we are lonely; we are depressed and anxious; and some of us are suicidal. I could not find myself between those lines. Although confronting my nonheterosexual orientation was not an easy and smooth process at all, it was not that destructive either. Once again, I felt that I did not belong and fit into the typical narrative of LGBTQ individuals. I was fat, fem, and a fag. Too much? Maybe.

My coming-out process went pretty smoothly. At the age of 15, I first came out to one of my best female friends at the time and she was completely indifferent about it, which provided me with the kind of reassurance I think I was looking for from her back then. Next in line was my mother. I was extremely anxious about the consequences of coming out to my mom. I had so many different scripts in mind, and none of them was even close to what really happened. I asked my mom to have dinner at a nice restaurant because there was something I needed to tell her. Hesitantly, I stuttered that I thought I was attracted to men. With a big smile she said: "I know, honey, I know." I did not expect it to be that easy. As always, my mom was my biggest supporter. I asked her to make the process of coming out a bit easier for me and tell my entire family about my nonheterosexual orientation, and so she did. Everything went pleasantly well. When I told my father that I was attracted to men, he was a bit shocked and said that now he has to deal with having two nonheterosexual kids. That was when I realized that my oldest brother is gay. I then came out to my close friends, all of whom were tremendously supportive. In general, I cannot recall any negative experience while coming out as nonheterosexual. From that moment on, I have been proudly living my life as a nonheterosexual person and am celebrating every aspect of it.

Too many times in my lifetime strangers have approached me to let me know that I have a beautiful face and gorgeous eyes, and that, if I really wanted to be a stunner, I should lose weight. This is not confined to me. If you are fat, people will focus on your face and ignore your body, as if it does not belong to you, or alternatively, overemphasize your shape, size, and weight. I have always found those comments to be offensive and inappropriate coming from strangers who have never even met me, but I never said anything in response. In fact, I did not know what to say, or rather, I agreed with them.

When I was 23 years old, I went to the supermarket deli to buy cheese for my sandwiches. I asked the vendor for a pound of Swiss cheese. He looked at me, smiling, and said: "It is a shame that you eat that much cheese. You are so beautiful, you could be a model . . . you just need to lose some weight." I was shocked. Never in my life would I have thought that a complete stranger whom I had never met would be that intrusive and rude. I took the cheese, ate my delicious sandwich, and for the first time in my life realized that from a very early age I had internalized people's opinions about me and my body. I accepted the conditioning that I have a beautiful face but a fat and repulsive body that cannot be attractive to anyone. I finally recognized how others' opinions about me and my body alienated me from my own body, sex appeal, and sexuality. Being well acquainted with self-hatred and the process of self-acceptance and self-love despite pervasive stigma and prejudice, I decided: no more of that crap. I declared a new beginning.

This is how my journey of self-love began. I decided that from that moment on I would deconstruct every negative opinion and conditioning I had internalized throughout the years and went on a journey of self-discovery. For the first time in my life, I started touching myself: my fat belly, my fat legs, my fat breast, my fat hips, and my fat ass. I stood naked in front of the mirror and discovered hidden parts of body that I have never seen before and revealed "new" features of my fat body. I followed every stretch mark I had proudly acquired through the hard work of being fat. I also rediscovered my fat folds and gained so much respect for every fat and flabby part of my body. I realized that having this type of body is a lifetime achievement and that I should be proud of it, every single part of it. If a person works hard at the gym to get the desired (not by me) "six-pack abs" and as a result feels free to show off his body, so can I. I worked hard and faced enough challenges in my life to get to the body I now have. With no hesitation, I can say that I love my beautiful self and my sexy body.

When you are constantly being pushed to the social margins, little by little you may feel forced to make yourself feel at home there. To feel like home, you have to furnish and design the place according to your unique taste. It was only then that I realized that my "otherness" was, in fact, my uniqueness. With the unconditional love and support of my family, I concentrated on healing myself by reframing my past experiences as special events that have formed my unique self. I abandoned any negative self-assessments and instead focused on self-love.

Working to overcome the hurdles of marginalization ignited my sensitivity to human suffering and passion for social change. I learned that having access to resources, such as social support and community involvement, may be the best way to mitigate the negative impact of marginalization and promote self-love. I embraced my uniqueness and became an ambassador of self-love, chiefly within the fat rights movement and the LGBTQ community. As an activist and a scholar, my main mission is to secure the necessary resources for fat and LGBTQ individuals to embrace their uniqueness, exercise self-love, and facilitate their personal growth and thriving. This is one way, I believe, we would reach a greater level of acceptance and respect within future generations for all fat and LGBTQ individuals.

In a world where the "war on obesity" is so rampant and pervasive, I am proud to publicly display my fat body. My body serves a resistance and symbol of protest against the widely spread fat-shaming discourse. Since the age of 23, when I first came out of the closet as a fat individual, I have been proud of my body. I am filled with joy to say that for my 29 years of living, I am now at my fattest and I LOVE IT! Here's to the 5F revolution.

19

"Fat Doesn't Crack": Exploring Youth Privilege in the Context of Fat

Lesleigh J. Owen

"Fat doesn't crack." I'd heard the phrase a hundred times before attending my first National Association for the Advancement of Fat Acceptance (NAAFA) convention. The phrase, meant to celebrate the wrinkle-free youthfulness of fat faces, always bothered me, but not with the sting of having experienced—or even having thought too hard about the implications of—ageism.

This all changed during the mid-aughts while I conducted research for my dissertation. My understanding of ageism, particularly as it intersects with sizeism, came in an interesting form: through experiencing youth privilege. Sure, I had known youth privilege my entire life, but it crystallized for me in the late summer of 2006. Perhaps it was because I was experiencing my world, my spaces, as a researcher rather than just a participant. Perhaps it was because I existed in a venue where the overwhelming burden of sizeism was temporarily, partially lifted. Whatever the reason, I grasped during that week in 2006 some of the many links between fatness and age, including how they coexist, why they threaten, and even some of their liberatory possibilities.

I adapted this chapter from a chapter of my dissertation, which I completed in 2008 after engaging in several years of research. For my dissertation, I employed four main research methodologies: participant journaling, interviews, ethnography, and autoethnography. For the first, I solicited almost 40 self-identified "fat" (or "large," "chubby," "big," "plus-size," "husky," and so on) participants and asked them to maintain body journals for several weeks or months.

From there, I advertised and asked several journalers for interviews as well as sought recommendations for interviewees. I tried very hard, and with mild success, to unearth male and nonwhite participants, since the persons most likely to respond to my ads were white women. Altogether, I interviewed the more than 100 interviewees in person and via e-mail, instant messaging, and telephone.

Finally, I engaged in what social researchers call "ethnography," or "participant observation." This method involves locating the researcher in the culture she or he wishes to study. I chose to participate in BBW (big, beautiful women) dance clubs and fat pride events. While my research notes from these experiences focus on other people, our surroundings, and the subcultures in general, I was surprised when many of them turned into somewhat extended journal entries for my own negotiations of the many meanings of "fat." Eventually, I had two sets of notes: my participant observation field notes (or ethnography) and my notes about my own life and inner workings (or my autoethnography). As Ellis, Adams, and Bochner note, "Autoethnography is an approach to research and writing that seeks to describe and systematically analyze personal experience in order to understand cultural experience."[1] Much of my discussion below includes information from my journalers and interviewees, but a great deal of it also comes from my research notes in the form of autoethnography.

I attended my first NAAFA annual convention in August 2006. I flew from Los Angeles to Boston all alone, nervous and exhilarated about submerging myself for several days in an atmosphere members of the local NAAFA chapter had described to me as "fairy-tale-like" and "all-encompassing" in its warmth and inclusiveness. The next several days were indeed shocking and surreal as I learned to readjust my definition of "average" body size and navigate an environment in which I was suddenly and explicitly a privileged member.

The following sections are direct excerpts from my research field notes; rather than summarize them and dilute their immediacy, I include them in their entirety.

NAAFA CONVENTION 2006

During the NAAFA Board announcements, someone said models were still needed for the vendor fashion show. Elsa told me I should model something at least once at a convention; she talks about her modeling experience all the time with some pride. I decided to volunteer, and they said they probably wouldn't use me; however, an hour later, I received a call from the fashion show organizer who told me to visit BBW Plus (a plus-size clothing vendor) to get a fitting. When I arrived in their hotel room, the vendors were somewhat dismayed to find I was a size 30 rather than a 32; I was too small for what they wanted modeled. Now *that's* a new experience! They finally hauled out a princess dress in my size and told me to model it. They also seemed quite pleased by my overall appearance.

Later on, as I was getting my hair professionally styled for the fashion show, another vendor approached me to model one outfit for her. I will never forget her reaction when she approached me; she looked surprised. She asked me how I was doing, and I cheerfully replied, "I'm lovely!" "Yes, you are," she said in surprise and delight. That was an enormous moment for me. I realized from both vendors' reactions (I'd already suspected, but this confirmed it for me) that I was a member of a privileged group. I am fat, yes, but I'm also young and White. In this group, I am closer to racist, ageist beauty ideals than many. This was a profound and extremely troubling insight for me, one that I agonized over and nurtured and pondered a long time.

How unusual, how sparkly, how deliciously weird to have the weight (ha ha!) of my fatness dismissed. In this place of empowerment, where we tried to topple anti-fat sentiments, I was merely average. My body type was the norm. With that out of the way, many of those who engaged with me showered with me attention and appreciation for my *relative* nearness to media beauty ideals (i.e., White, young, long hair, somewhat tall, well dressed, able-bodied, seemingly heterosexual).

While I'm discussing it, I may as well confess to feeling very odd [about this recognition of my privilege, thrown as it was into stark relief by the dismissal of my normally devalued fat body]. I struggle every single day of my life to keep my head high, meet everyone's eyes, project power, and recognize my beauty in others' eyes whether or not *they* see it. I fight others' hatred and fear of my body and try to demonstrate, through my confidence and my performance of a traditional kind of (seeming) heterofemininity, that I am more than what others would reduce me to. But in NAAFA I got my very first taste of what it might be like to have beauty privilege without internally manufacturing it. Beauty in this context was more than a mindset, more than a mental and physical space I painfully carved for myself out of others' hostilities, more than keeping my chin up and my back straight. Beauty was a privilege I had *without doing anything*. In comparison to the other [attendees], most of whom were older than me and some of whom were not energetic and able-bodied, I was among the physically privileged. I have never, ever before experienced this. I saw my privilege reflected as "beauty" in others' eyes; I felt their awareness of me as a privileged person. I never felt resentment from anyone, but I did feel their eyes following me all the time.

This was one of the scariest and most exhilarating feelings I have ever experienced. On the one hand, I saw it as a matter of privilege, and as I always tell my students, privilege always comes at the expense of someone else; it cannot exist without its twin, oppression. My privilege came at others' expense.

However, and here's the kicker: *I also wanted to keep that feeling forever.* I'm ashamed to say this, but I can't deny it. I would never want anyone to hurt as a result of my own privilege, and I loathe oppression in all forms. In spite of this, though, I felt myself struggling to maintain my privileges, to highlight them, to add them to my overall repertoire of fabulousness.

Every day I appeared at workshops, I was well-dressed. Even though I seldom wear make-up (well, except my lipstick, of course), and rarely don mascara, *I wore them every single day I attended the NAAFA Convention.* I did my hair in creative and attractive styles that flowed down my back (even though I hate wearing my hair down!). I kept lipstick with me at all times and reapplied it often. I eagerly posed for pictures (okay, I always eagerly pose for pictures). I felt like the same happy, enthusiastic Lesleigh, but I walked through corridors and sat in chairs with a presence that I don't usually have. Normally, I am aware of my body, aware of its size and others' awareness of it. I often feel— or imagine I do—their judgment of me, their unfriendly eyes, their fear and loathing of what I represent. As a result, I enact a type of beauty in my everyday life that thumbs its nose at the world. I create my own beauty and defiantly occupy it. I live my body aware of others' disdain but confidently swinging my hips and coloring my lips red as a statement of femmey beauty, physicality, and pride. At NAAFA, this defiant performance of self-love was unnecessary, and I felt what beauty means to those who are [normally] nearer the ideals than I. In this new context, with its different reference points, I was nearer the ideal and aware of myself in entirely new ways.

The experience helped me gain new insights into my own sources of privilege. It's easy to focus on being an oppressed fat woman and forget that I'm also a fat, White, young, able-bodied woman who dresses femininely and enacts a very familiar kind of (apparent) heterofemininity. No wonder skinny and young (etc.) women fear losing their sources of privilege; once you have it, you start investing in it, start seeing the approval and envy in others' eyes and feeling validated because of it. Unlike my everyday life, in which I fight fiercely for self-respect and a sense of beauty and loving physicality, this experience, these feelings, are merely handed to some women. It's easy to feel good when one is adored; it's so much more difficult to be the source of one's own validation and recognition. I felt this when I noticed myself using make-up every single day, which I *never* do, as well as letting my annoying hair swing free (in, as Oprah has discussed, its very White and idealized way), which is unheard of. I suddenly had an investment in media-defined [and heterofeminine] beauty ideals, which, in this context, I all but achieved. *This is something I had never known I could experience.* [For an expanded analysis of beauty privilege, including the difficulty in achieving it and the subsequent terror of losing it, see Frost's discussion of Tseelon.][2]

... I have to wonder if some of us fatties who have politicized our bodies and recognized beauty as a social construct are even happier than average or smaller-sized women. As Naomi Wolf says in *The Beauty Myth*, old women fear younger women for their privilege and judgment and younger women fear older women as symbols of what they will eventually lose.[3] This keeps women generationally separated. As it is, I fear thin women because of their privilege, judgment, and their pro-jected self-hatred, and I know most thin women fear us fatties as remind-ers of what they [can] become. Fat or thin, we all feel separated, isolated, and unhappy. Those of us who turn this issue into a public and political one find a community of others like us and feel less alone and more ener-gized. Imagine being an isolated, fearful skinny woman who thinks she's the *only* one who obsesses over [getting fat and losing her thin privilege]. It's the emperor's new clothes.

Fat women become a scapegoat for this universal body hatred, but we all feel it. At the convention, I felt fear for the first time at the prospect of losing my youth. Privilege is such a double-edged sword; it both empowers and enslaves. Skinny women, for example, can't imagine the horror of being fat like me, but they're already living their own night-mares, chained to a beauty ideal of thinness that constantly threatens them with exclusion and shame. Likewise, I can't imagine how terrible it must be to have ageism heaped on top of the sizeism, homophobia, and sexism I know all-too-well, but the heretofore unacknowledged fear of this inevitability kept me slathering on the mascara and putting extra bounces in my step.

NAAFA CONVENTION 2007

While Daphne ran the fashion show, Rachel and I submitted ourselves to the cattle roundup of models. All of us potentials gathered into a cen-tral herd and awaited clothing vendors to brand us as their models. I was unpleasantly and grumpily reminded of sixth grade gym class, in which I was always picked last for teams. But I wasn't picked last here. Gina Madison, manager of Divine Curves [in Southern California], who also apparently designs clothing, immediately chose Rachel and me as her fashion show models because we were "young and vivacious." I tried to feel flattered but instead felt annoyed and disgusted. Gina's ageism reminded me that even as this is supposedly a safe place for people of size, other cultural hierarchies remain. . . .

[During the fashion show,] I modeled a blue and yellow bikini as well as a short brown sundress with skulls sporting pink bows, a red flowered sundress, and an ankle-length blue dress with a green shrug. I had a tremendous time modeling and being an enormous ham onstage; I danced, shimmied, fanned myself, and was otherwise saucy. I had a divine (pun kind of intended) time, but I never really lost that nagging feeling that I was such a hit onstage and with the vendors not merely because I'm a drama queen and an enthusiastic activist but because I'm young and White with long brown hair.

. . . Hierarchies are somewhat different in this community than in others. As a person of size, I often feel marginalized, dismissed, rejected in mainstream culture. Here, size isn't a big deal; in fact, I didn't even feel that smaller women were more privileged, although perhaps others feel that way. (Some would argue the opposite, in fact.) Also, I estimate that probably 85–90% of NAAFA Convention attendees are White, which means I'm not abnormally privileged but instead part of the invisible, taken-for-granted, privileged racial group.

The biggest, most profound privilege I experienced was in regards to my age. Other NAAFAns constantly commented on my "beauty." Granted, I like to think of myself as a cutie, but I have a suspicion others' effusive praise had less to do with my inherent physical charms and more to do with my youth, Whiteness, ability, and enactment of a very nonthreatening femininity. Would Taylor and Tara, two (in my mind) gorgeous but butch fat activists, although both White and a few years younger than me, be considered as "pretty" [and celebration-worthy]?

While we were there, Daphne, Rachel, and I hung out with the other young, childless women; we formed a cadre that socialized together. Although my racial and other privileges remained a gentle hum, I experienced my youth privilege like a shout throughout convention. . . . Viewing the elderly as an oppressed *minority* is a trick of cowardice: we are all old; for some of us it just doesn't yet show.[4]

I talked with a woman the other day—she's . . . a fat activist—and she said, "You're Lauren?!" and I said "Yeah." She said, "You have such a baby face!" I felt extremely uncomfortable because I knew she was saying that out of envy and because she was saying implicitly that I'm prettier. Ugly and old are as synonymous as ugly and fat. (Lauren, personal interview)

Like white, male, or any other privilege, youth privilege is contextual. For example, finding my 18-year-old frosh students blinking silently at me as I discuss the Clarence Thomas and Anita Hill debacle, I can sometimes feel quite embarrassingly unhip and dated (terms that have become almost synonymous). However, at NAAFA conventions, I felt youthful, spry, hip. Other, older attendees thanked me profusely for coming, addressed comments about the "next generation of activists" my way, and praised my vitality. I felt invincible.

I am interested in locating youth privilege in the context of sizeism— more specifically, within my and others' experiences with our fat. Below, I divide into three categories overlapping, contradictory, sometimes constructive moments when fat and old intersect.

Discussing fatness without addressing its intersections with aging is inconceivable to me. After all, sizeism and ageism as forms of oppression have many similarities, being mapped arbitrarily onto bodies as they are *and* looming as a constant fear (or eventuality) in our popular consciousness. I would argue that advertising, particularly for women, focuses heavily (if often in reverse, i.e., by excluding them) these two "preventable" or minimizable bodily conditions, creating an especially pernicious haze of fear and dread around them. According to Wolf in *The Beauty Myth*, the two greatest fears in our culture are weight and age.[5] While I don't agree they're the *most* feared, I do agree that fatness and age loom in the minds of everyone, threatening them with their potential inevitability.

In addition, and quite simply, the two topics seem highly connected since, like nonwhite ones, older bodies are often bigger ones.[6] As a result, fat elders embody two sets of echoing rhetorics around body capabilities: fat and older bodies, we hear, are sick, potentially disabled, unproductive, and in need of monitoring and regulation.[7]

As disability activists say, "able-bodied" persons can more accurately be described as "temporarily-abled,"[8] a fact that often becomes more salient to us as we age. Similarly, many persons are "temporarily thin," since many currently thin persons are only one accident, one medical condition, or X number of years away from fatness. While certainly not simultaneous or synonymous, fatness, old age, and disabilities sometimes occur concurrently, both in the ways we talk about them and in their actualities.

Is it because of these overlaps that NAAFA and the fat pride movement in Southern California find themselves populated by women (and a few men) in our forties through sixties? After all, metabolic rates are higher during youth, and for younger women, menopause as a source of weight gain is not yet a consideration. Why focus on their fat when they still benefit from the youth worship permeating our culture?[9] Fat youths may experience the stigma of sizeism, but like some working-class white men who embrace a kind of hypermasculinity in part to compensate for their lack of class privilege,[10] so do some young persons revel in their youth privilege while trying to minimize or eliminate (through dieting and, as Goffman would call it, "covering")[11] their stigmatized fatness. In short, younger persons, who occupy a highly favorable body type in terms of age, may well choose to highlight their youth (or, as the title of this chapter suggests, the physical appearance of which) and minimize their fatness. As Jacquelyn, a 38-year-old, white, self-described feminist commented during her interview with me,

> At a younger age, I felt that feminine power, that conventionally attractive, feminine power. . . . I don't feel like I have that sexual cachet anymore. That's a big change for me. . . . There's this immediate sense between men and me that they think I'm a bitch and I think they're full of shit and we both know this about each other. That never happened when I was younger. Even though I may not have been trying to work it, I was benefiting from that privilege. It seems like there's a combination of invisibility and dismissiveness now about a lot of strange men when I have to interact with them that wouldn't have happened before.

Likewise, Pamela, a 37-year-old, white academic in religious and fat studies, discussed with some dismay in her journal her increasing dissatisfaction with her body. During our interview, she pointed out the greatest source of her newfound self-consciousness: a line down her forearm, dividing lean from fat. We both laughed, and she acknowledged that her increasing awareness of the "flaws" of her body "is about aging and about how weight settles differently as you get older and you get things like wrinkles. And how some of those ways that fat is settling on me right now, at 37, are making me feel like a dowdy old lady." Although a fat studies academic and advocate for fat rights, Pamela had always felt much more comfortable with her fat body before it started showing signs of aging.

Another example occurred in Kate's interview. Kate, who is 30 years old, white, and blond, told me she almost exclusively dates thin, older, working-class men. She likes flirting with and dating older, working-class men, she told me, because they seem more "open-minded" about fat women and also because the possibility of a meaningful relationship seems "less real." Interesting to me was her choice to date older men almost exclusively. While certainly she may simply enjoy more mature conversations, I couldn't help but wonder, especially given her comments about "less real" relationships, whether she dates older men because, although she is fat, she brings her youth to the dating market as a source of privilege for both participants.

Lauren, the women whose quote appears earlier in the chapter, recounted a similar story. She dated for more than 2 years a man 18 years her senior. Not only did he fetishize her fatness as a symbol of sexual excess, but he also introduced her to his friends as "my 22-year-old girlfriend." It was a simple trade-off, she told me. "[My boyfriend] benefited from my age and I benefited from having a man in my life and making my mom happy. 'See, Mom? I'm not thin or straight, but I can do what I'm, what good girls are, supposed to.'"

Somewhat contrarily, as least seemingly so, is the number of fat research participants who told me they have gained a greater understanding of and affinity with their bodies. In fact, a large number of my older interviewees told me they felt more at home with their older bodies as they learned to free themselves from the rat race of pursuing unachievable, young, "beautiful" feminine ideals. Danica, Bonnie, Joel, Caeryn, Amelia, Daphne, and Julie all waxed poetic about their relatively newfound comfort and appreciation for their older bodies. As their opportunities for youth privilege diminished, they found themselves less and less inclined to pursue it. Or, as 50-year-old, white Caeryn phrased it, "We don't have to worry about that shit anymore!"

But is this really a contradiction, or might it be a loophole in institutional oppression? In spite of the crushing weight of sizeism and ageism, the invisibility of fat and older—let alone older fat—persons in popular culture, might fat and older persons have found a way to wiggle around, or at least negotiate, some forms of freedom from cultural oppression? Cultural sizeism and ageism have rendered many fat and older persons (again, depending on their identity sets) less capable of achieving media-defined physical ideals. And isn't there a certain kind of wonderful in that?

In my research notes above, I ponder whether I'm happier with my body than most thin women, since I'm aware of it, invested in it, politicized around it. Likewise, just by virtue of having fat, I have already failed to enact a diminutive, heterosexual kind of femininity. Away from the privilege game, I find I can relax and enjoy other pursuits. I feel free, or at least freer. As I have written elsewhere:

> Another consideration is the ubiquitous term: "letting oneself go." This is used constantly in magazines, on daytime talk shows, in warnings from friends and parents to new brides and college frosh (of the feminine sort, of course!). What does this mean? Explicitly, of course, it is a warning not to succumb to bodily appetites and risk bulking up and becoming visually unconsumable. Implicitly, however, "letting oneself go" implies gaining freedom from some kind of imprisonment. As Tisdale writes, "The fat persons' character flaw is a lack of narcissism. She's let herself go" (2005: 5). "Letting oneself go seems to me to imply not only a physical looseness but perhaps also a rather scary escape from the dictates of oppressive beauty ideals" (Hartley, 2001). Is that another reason why fat persons seem so threatening: because we are seen as having freed

ourselves from the cutthroat rat race of striving for unachievable beauty and gender ideals?[12]

Like fat persons, haven't older ones "let themselves go"? Might there be a delicious freedom in knowing one can never measure up to arbitrary beauty ideals? While I don't think every older or fat person perceives the devaluation of his or her body as a freedom, it does seem obvious to me that there exists at least some opportunity for an escape from the seemingly endless pursuit of bodily ideals. After all, I imagine I wouldn't have had to highlight and guard my youth privilege at the NAAFA convention had I not been able to taste it in the first place.

Privilege, while bestowing benefits, also hurts and constrains. Even a little bit of it can make its recipients feel invested in the system that allows them one step up the ladder of privilege. Might those who subconsciously wallow in their privilege, who fiercely protect it, feel more confined, more tied to an unequal, hierarchical system in which everyone scrambles to climb one more ladder rung, than those who will never fit on the ladder or who have been kicked off it?

This is not to glorify the oppression of older and fat persons, of course. I am merely thinking through the relief many of my older, fat interviewees expressed at "not worrying about that shit." Might this be one of the many reasons why younger and thinner people sometimes demonstrate a fear of and anger about aging and fatness disproportionate to mere years lived or additional pounds? Instead of supposedly hating us because we represent ill health (something both older and fat persons hear constantly), might much of their rage really lie in knowing many of us have "let ourselves go"? Might some of that seething anger stem from knowing we have escaped the unsteady ladder of privilege and are living perfectly livable lives without vying for the hardest bodies, the fewest wrinkles, the random beauty points? We have "failed" and through our failure have gained a chance at freedom. Fat and older bodies threaten this system of inequalities by refusing to bolster it.

I am 39 years old now—7 years older than the grad student who attended her first NAAFA convention. I am still told "You sure don't look your age!" and regarded as one of the younger and hipper instructors at the university at which I teach. While I am pretty far beyond what's cool in pop culture, I certainly don't know what it means to find realistic depiction of persons of my age almost completely absent from mainstream media.

In spite of all this, I feel the slipping of my privilege. I hear it in the panic in my friends' and partner's voices when they discuss their birthdays. I see it in the aggressive absence on billboards and in magazines of bodies featuring my crow's feet and festive "hair tinsel." As someone who is approaching 40,

I know popular culture doesn't represent my lifestyle, my desires. Whether or not I currently "look it," I'm getting older; I feel my privilege drifting further and further away.

As a lifelong person of size, I know a little bit about finding oneself marginalized in popular media, referred to in terms that imply weakness and debility, avoided for fear of contagion, regarded as a threat to body ideals and constructions of "beauty," silently encouraged to stay home because the world isn't built for my kind of physicality, derided for supposedly being sick and putting too much strain on the health care industry, hated for reminding people what may very well happen to them. This is not to say my ageism and sizeism are identical but to recognize the many points of overlap.

I am fat. Defined as they are by social institutions, I can only partially and conditionally occupy categories of health, beauty, and value. Interestingly, it was only when my fatness became neutral that I gained a greater understanding of what it meant to fit into these cultural categories and become invested in them.

I experience youth privilege; however, it is a different youth privilege than a thinner woman might experience. Outside of NAAFA, for example, my fat youth will likely not qualify as beautiful or healthy. How can a fat woman be beautiful? Healthy? Able-bodied? Yet because of my youth, I can still find a toehold in these categories. I may be fat, but I am young(ish), energetic and able-bodied, white, and cisgender. On ratemyprofessors.com, I have a decent hotness rating (don't get me started on why students can rate their professors' hotness). In 10 years, I expect this rating will diminish in direct proportion to the blossoming of my wrinkles and the explosion of my hair tinsel.

My fatness mitigates, informs, and is informed by my relative youth. I am privileged, but "fat and young" carries with it different cultural messages and privileges than "thin or young" or, of course, "fat and old." Outside NAAFA, where my fatness becomes neutralized, I am a relatively young person of size living in a sexist, ageist culture. Being fat hurts; it certainly affects my youth privilege. That said, my relative youth and other identities still allow me to cast lots in the competitive game of privilege, where there are definite winners and losers. Unfortunately, these are games whose rules constrain, hurt, and pit us in opposition to one another. Depending on my context, I am winner of this game. Loser. Something in-between. It is a game I don't wish to play but that, regardless of my wishes, I must learn to negotiate. I may not enjoy this game, but it remains rooted in institutions and as such is larger and more entrenched than one not-so-little sociologist.[13]

The game of inequalities may not need me to keep it going, but I will still try to minimize my participation as much as possible. After all, fat may crack, and isn't it wonderful to imagine what will spill forth when it does?

NOTES

1. Carolyn Ellis, Tony E. Adams, and Arthur P. Bochner, "Autoethnography: An Overview," *Forum: Qualitative Social Research* 12, no. 1 (2011), http://www.qualitative-research.net/index.php/fqs/article/view/1589/3095.

2. Liz Frost, *Young Women and the Body: A Feminist Sociology* (New York: Palgrave, 2001), 46.

3. Naomi Wolf, *The Beauty Myth: How Images of Beauty Are Used against Women* (New York: Morrow, 1991), 130.

4. Wendy Chapkis, *Beauty Secrets: Women and the Politics of Appearance* (Boston: South End Press, 1986), 15, emphasis mine.

5. Wolf, *The Beauty Myth*, 134.

6. Chris Shilling, *The Body and Social Theory*, 2nd ed. (London: Sage, 2003), 116; Bryan S. Turner, "The Discourse of Diet," in *The Body: Social Process and Cultural Theory*, ed. Mike Featherstone, Mike Hepworth, and Bryan S. Turner (London: Sage, 1991), 161.

7. W. Charisse Goodman, *The Invisible Woman: Confronting Weight Prejudice in America* (Carlsbad, CA: Gürez Books, 1995), 23; Sondra Solovay, "Now You See Me, Now You Don't," in *Scoot Over, Skinny: The Fat Nonfiction Anthology*, ed. Donna Jarrell and Ira Sukrungruang (Orlando, FL: Harcourt, 2005), 104.

8. Shirley Castelnuovo and Sharon R. Guthrie, *Feminism and the Female Body: Liberating the Amazon Within* (Boulder, CO: L. Rienner, 1998).

9. *The Merchants of Cool*, PBS Video (Boston: WGBH Educational Foundation, 2001).

10. Michael Kimmel, *Angry White Men: American Masculinity at the End of an Era* (New York: Nation Books, 2013), 33.

11. Erving Goffman, *Stigma: Notes on the Management of Spoiled Identity* (New York: Simon and Schuster, 1963), 6.

12. Lesleigh Owen, "Tightening Up Loose Bodies and Morals: Dieting Away the Sin," *The Body as a Site of Discrimination* (2009), http://www.bodydiscrimination.com/.

13. Robert Alun Jones, *Emile Durkheim: An Introduction to Four Major Works* (Beverly Hills, CA: Sage, 1986), 63.

20

Tales of a Cyborg: A Fat Crip Assemblage

Candice Buss

January 16, 2013, was supposed to be a rebirth for me. It was supposed to signal my transition from "broken spine" to "cyborg athlete/dancer." My spinal fusion was supposed to fix my persnickety slipped lumbar vertebra that was gnawing on the nerves related to my legs and part of my pelvis. It was supposed to get me back to the gleeful kinesiologist that I am, the one that studies joyful physical activity regardless of body size or dis/ability.

I was in surgery for five and a half hours that Wednesday morning. It was the first week of classes in the second semester of the first year of my doctoral program, and I was going under the knife for a surgery with a severely mixed success rate. I needed to have two vertebrae fused together with four titanium screws, two small rods, a plastic cage, and some cadaver bone to stabilize a grade 2 spondylolysthesis (medical term for a slipped vertebra) that was causing nerve and spinal cord damage. Without the surgery, I would continue to lose function in my lower body. I would be in more and more pain, be in need of more and stronger prescription pain medication, and require more and more trips to the emergency room to get my pain-induced high blood pressure under control. To borrow a term from Donna Haraway,[1] I needed to become a cyborg with these implants.

So much hope in this procedure. I was sick of doctors treating me as if my pain was related to a combination of fatness and inactivity. I was sick of spending eight hours trying to explain to emergency room doctors that my blood pressure is usually borderline low versus incredibly high. I needed to be able to think clearly to be able to be a competent and productive scholar of kinesiology and public health. Most importantly to me, I wanted to be back to my athletic pursuits. Before my spine started compressing the nerves to my lower body, I was an avid power lifter, bicyclist, triathlete, runner, semiprofessional belly dancer, and whatever else my heart wanted to try. What I really wanted was my adventurous spirit back, something that chronic pain and nerve damage took away from me because of a reliance on canes, crutches, wheelchairs, and opioid pain medication.

There are many assumptions placed on the fat body. Poststructuralist theorists would say that the body is a text that can be read, and the fat body in the twenty-first century is read as being lazy, sedentary, overconsuming, disgusting, and in medical settings treatment noncompliant. The disabilities I was born with, despite biomedical correlations with fatness, have never exempted me from these stereotypes. My fatness has always prompted doctors to tell me to eat less and move more, even when eating disordered as a gymnast teen or when doing triathlons and distance cycling. If I could prove that I wasn't lazy, I was read as a liar.

Somehow, despite people not believing my activity levels, I kept putting myself out in the public eye in this "before" time. Despite college boys mooing at my fat butt bike commuting, despite difficulties finding triathlon clothing for racing, despite having trouble finding dancewear for round bodies, despite running stores insisting that I ought to be looking at walking shoes instead of running shoes . . . despite society's expectations of what I ought to be doing, I loved moving my body. I loved pushing my body in novel ways and trying new things. My prefracture life was like a personification of Daft Punk's song "Harder Better Faster Stronger" because I wanted to see what my little garden gnome-shaped body could accomplish.

Both my pre- and postoperative medical care was compromised because many doctors and nursing staff made assumptions about my body that could have been devastating, and did in fact lead to several traumatic experiences. In the month before my surgery, my partner brought me to the emergency department of the local hospital an average of once per week because of pain so severe I was having trouble breathing. As a part of the triage process, the staff would take my blood pressure and immediately assume that a systolic blood pressure of 170 was normal for me because of my fat body. Whether or not high blood pressure was a part of my body's norm, no matter my size (which at a body mass index of 50 is big enough that bariatric surgery is frequently suggested), my individual human nature was repeatedly taken from me.

The day after my spinal fusion surgery, I dealt with a couple of very pissed-off people because I literally could not move myself because of 10/10 pain that wasn't alleviated by one shot of morphine (and neither the nurses nor my surgeon's assistant would give me anything else . . . no drip, no self-push button device, no other medication . . . I was ignored when I told them that the pain management was inadequate). They wanted an X-ray but visibly did not want to try to transfer the fat person from the hospital bed to the X-ray table. My severe dislike for being carried is magnified while six people transfer my 250-pound freshly cyborg body from the hospital bed to the X-ray table and back again. I stay quiet and cry not only throughout the procedure but as I wait for a nursing assistant to roll me back to my room on the orthopedic floor.

Sleep evades me for the entire three-day stay at the hospital and I refuse to call the hospital staff to help me shift in bed or to use the bathroom. I cry off and on, worrying about being mistreated further because of my body size.

I'm at my three-month surgical evaluation with my surgeon. He is visibly disappointed when I tell him that I still need to be on narcotic medications because of moderate to severe pain. He's disappointed that I started physical therapy (PT) "late" per his usual surgical schedule because I insisted on seeing the physical therapist that I saw before surgery. Even though he doesn't say it, he has before. His face tells me that once I get through PT, I need to be on a diet and exercise plan. I'm being read through the lens of the obesity epidemic rhetoric and I'm frustrated. He used to call me "his dancer" and would ask how "his dancer" was doing. When he said this, I hadn't seriously danced for a few years but being "his dancer" made me feel like he was committed to giving me my pre-spine fracture life back. Perhaps he didn't believe that I was a fat dancer and athlete.

If I could become thin, I would be fixed. By magic. Magical nerve and spine healing that would allow me to completely feel my legs and run and leap and spin.

I'm knee deep in the rehab process with a body that remains undeniably queer and malformed. I'm still physically and mentally crippled by pain, by balance problems, by proprioception issues. To maintain "normal" posture involves an incredible amount of mental fortitude. Standing upright without a cane or crutch is a balancing act akin to some yoga poses. Walking without wobbling requires concentration. My physical therapist understands as she underwent a spine fusion procedure in her neck. She reminds me that spine surgery is no guarantee of a pain-reduced life. She listens to me when I talk about my surgeon's fat phobia and how it impacts my recovery thought process. Because she's never once talked about my body in a negative way (neither my fat nor my painful cyborg bits of titanium holding my lower spine together), I trust her guidance.

Because I'm a naturally active person, the real point of PT seems to be to convince me that the surgery wasn't a failure. I'm told that the first purpose of PT is to get me stronger so I will be able to stand, sit, and walk as safely and as pain-free as possible so I can work and have a full and productive life. As I still need to take strong prescription pain killers to be able to endure PT, I realize that PT is really only helping me perform a semblance of abledness. She tells me that even in the best-case scenario I will have pain flare-ups that may incapacitate me. On a masochistic whim, I decide to ask her if I will ever be able to dance or lift weights again. Her face falls and I know in my heart that I don't want to hear what's going to come out of her mouth.

I'm struggling with my identity as an athlete, as a kinesiologist, and as someone who believes that joyful physical activity is a human rights and justice issue. I feel like I'm 15 again, questioning my place in the world at large. I have this body that contains a brain that wants to move vigorously, to feel "The Burn" that the aerobics videos of the 1980s would espouse, but I can't. I can't dance in the way I want to, and now I have permanent weight-lifting restrictions that will no longer allow me to pick up a standard unloaded barbell (40-pound restriction; a standard barbell is 45 pounds). Who am I if I can't say that I'm a physically strong person anymore? Do I continue to say that I used to be able to back squat more than 175 pounds? What happens to the fat athlete who can't find accessible athletic endeavors?

As I piece these memories together, it's been almost 10 months since surgery. Because of maltreatment that I attribute mostly to my body size, I still have flashbacks from when I woke up from the surgery or from other parts of my three-day hospital stay. Sometimes I wake up in the middle of the night in a cold sweat remembering the moment when I emerged from the anesthetic haze. It was the moment that the quantitative malarkey of the 1–10 pain scale exploded. In that moment, all I could think about was pain. It was my cyborg rebirth. Much like the squalling infant newly emerged from the womb, I emerged from the cocoon of anesthesia flailing and wailing with only the ability to vaguely move my head and my limbs. My previous surgeries were unlike this experience. I felt raw, exposed, and scared, and those memories are intimately tied with society's expectations of the fat patient.

One day I hope that a person's body size will not be equated with signifiers of treatment incompliance. One day I hope that I will hear of other fat people experiencing life-altering surgeries that are not filled with assumptions and stereotypes. I will continue to hope for the day in which a fat athlete or dancer can be treated with equity and justice in medical settings as thinner active people are treated.

NOTE

1. Donna J. Haraway, "A Cyborg Manifesto: Science, Technology, and Socialist-Feminism in the Late Twentieth Century," in *Simians, Cyborgs, and Women: The Reinvention of Nature* (New York: Routledge, 1991), 149–81.

About the Editor and Contributors

THE EDITOR

RAGEN CHASTAIN is a trained researcher, three-time national champion dancer, and marathoner who writes and speaks full-time about self-esteem, body image, and health. Author of the blog *www.DancesWithFat.org* and the book *Fat: The Owner's Manual*, Ragen's writing has also been published in forums including the Calgary Herald, Democratic Underground, and Jezebel.com. Her work has been translated into multiple languages and her blog has readers on all seven continents. She is the body image and women's health blogger for NBCs iVillage and a columnist for *Ms. Fit* magazine. A leading activist in the Health at Every Size and size acceptance movements, Ragen passionately speaks for people of size and against the ill-conceived war on obesity. Ragen has recently spoken at universities and corporations around the country and is a feature interviewee in the documentaries *America the Beautiful 2: The Thin Commandments*, released by Warner Brothers in 2011, *A Stage for Size*, released 2013, and Ragen's *MORE Cabaret*, 2014. Ragen led the organization that raised more than $20,000 in eight days and put up six billboards and 10 bus shelter ads in Atlanta to counter a fat-shaming billboard campaign, and the Skinny Minnie petition, which garnered over 150,000 signatures and resulted in substantial changes to a promotion by Barney's and Disney.

THE CONTRIBUTORS

NADAV (NADIVA) ANTEBI is a proud fat PhD student in the Departments of Sociomedical Sciences and Psychology at Columbia University. They earned their BA in behavioral sciences in Tel-Aviv-Yaffo Academic College and their MA in human development from Cornell University. Their main line of research focuses on the positive aspects of stigmatized identities with a particular focus on LGBTQ and fat communities. For more than a decade, they have been working with LGBTQ populations in both community and research settings and is excited about integrating theory and research into real-life practice. Nadav believes that fat is fierce and self-love is fabulous.

KATE BROWNE is an English studies doctoral student at Illinois State University specializing in women's life writing and the lives of circus women. She plans to write her dissertation on autobiographical narratives of body size with an enthusiastic chapter on "sideshow fat ladies."

CANDICE BUSS is currently a doctoral student studying the sociology of physical activity. She lives with her partner in North Carolina along with two cats and a fish. In her spare time, she dances as much as she can and enjoys being a rad fattie gimp.

JUDI RICHARDSON/JOSEPHINE CRANBERRY passed away shortly after her piece for the anthology was finished. She died surrounded by her friends and she will continue to be missed. Many benefited from her life of activism, including some who never knew her. We all owe her a great debt of gratitude.

After a childhood in rural northern Minnesota, the author moved to Minneapolis to attend the University of Minnesota where she earned a bachelor's degree in 1967 with a major in journalism and a minor in history. In 1968, she moved to Delaware with her newlywed Air Force husband and earned teaching credentials in night classes while teaching second grade full-time. She moved to San Diego, California, in 1971 where she worked as a substitute teacher, temporary office worker, and Avon lady. Finally, she found full-time work as an eligibility worker, got a divorce, and progressed to quality control analyst, eligibility supervisor, and then appeals representative. While working full-time during the day, she attended law school at night and, in 1980, she earned a juris doctorate from Western State, now Jefferson Law University, and became a member of the California State Bar. She was on law review, authored an article on women and crime, and edited other articles for the publication. Following law school, she volunteered for various feminist groups including the Feminist Credit Union. She worked as a temporary hearing officer for the state of California, got a permanent job as an attorney, first for Legal Aid and then back to the state, and was appointed an administrative law judge in 1990.

The author became active in the size acceptance movement around 1988. She attended several conventions and retreats, put on workshops, participated in pickets of antifat businesses, marched to support the cause, and partied hearty at the dances. She was a member of size acceptance groups such as Mor2Luv, NAAFA, and the Size Diversity Task Force. She was one of the founding mothers of the Size Acceptance For Empowerment (SAFE) organization. Until her passing the author continued to work on planning, writing newsletters and providing leadership to implement activities that have grown well beyond the initial scope of retreats and swims for fat people. SAFE is in its 14th year. She tried not to volunteer for anything else.

In her final years Judi devoted her time to occasional Pro Tem judge work, writing, lots of reading, her cats, her man, crafting, and her patio garden, as well as her aforementioned involvement in the size acceptance movement.

DR. E-K DAUFIN is an educator, feminist minister, social activist performance artist, belly dancer, fine artist, EFT practitioner, *Love Your Body; Love Yourself* workshops founder, and *Health at Every Size Journal* columnist who earns a living as a professor of communication at Alabama State University. She earned a PhD in mass communication and film from The Ohio State University. Blog: http://daufination .blogspot.com. Home page: http://home.earthlink.net/~ekdaufin.

NANCY ELLIS-ORDWAY is a psychotherapist with 30 years of experience, specializing in treating eating disorders, body image issues, stress, anxiety, depression, and relationship issues. She offers individual, couple, and family therapy through her private practice in Jefferson City, Missouri. In addition to a master's of social work degree from Washington University, she has completed the advanced psychodynamic psychotherapy training program at the St. Louis Psychoanalytic Institute. She has previously written chapters for three books, as well as numerous articles for professional and general publications. She teaches professional continuing education programs in self-care, safety awareness for social workers, and applying Health at Every Size principles in psychotherapy. She is currently a doctoral candidate in health education and promotion at the University of Missouri.

KRISTEN A. HARDY is a doctoral candidate in social and political thought at York University, Toronto, Canada. Her work explores relations between systems of power and the constitution of marginalized subjects, with a focus on embodiment and pathologization in science, medicine, and other sociocultural spheres. Her research interests include the role of affect in the development of scientific cultures, the historical negotiation of human-nonhuman boundaries, and the constitution of fatness and fat bodies as socially and medically salient entities.

REBECCA D. HARRIS is a visual artist and independent researcher based in Launceston, UK. After gaining a first-class honors degree in fine art from Plymouth College of Art, she went on to complete a master's degree at Plymouth University in contemporary art practice. She has presented research papers and exhibited, in both solo and group shows, nationally within the UK.

RORY E. KRAFT JR. is assistant professor of philosophy at York College of Pennsylvania. His primary areas of work are in ethics (theoretical and applied) and philosophy with children. He earned a PhD from Michigan State, an MA from American University, and a BA from Arizona State—all in philosophy. He is editor of *Questions: Philosophy for Young People*, an annual journal dedicated to philosophy by, for, and with precollege students, and is treasurer of the American Association of Philosophy Teachers. He is married and has two children.

DR. LORI DON LEVAN is a graduate of Teachers College, Columbia University, New York, and holds an EdD in art education. She holds an MS in administration and supervision with a visual arts focus from Bank Street College of Education, New York, and a Parson's School of Design certificate. Her BFA (with K–12 art teaching certification) is from Wilkes University, Pennsylvania. She has taught all levels of art to young people and adults in a variety of settings and has devoted her life to the teaching of art and related subjects. "I truly believe that the act of making art is a special way of creating meaning in this world and that doing so gives us experiences that have unique qualities that can't be learned in any other way." She has also taught courses on the college level to undergraduates and graduate students with artistic themes that connect to women's studies, oral history, art education, outsider art, and visual culture. Dr. Levan is an active artist using photography, mixed media, and installation to explore issues concerning the body and beauty, memories lost and found, and the nature of the photographic image. She has shown her work in many venues including galleries in New York City and the surrounding region. Dr. Levan is a feminist and a fat activist and is a scholar supporting the emerging field of fat studies. Her work in this area has supported research that intersects with the arts, humanities, and sciences that calls into question assumed perceptions of fatness as they relate to the sociocultural landscape in the United States and beyond.

IRENE MCCALPHIN is a queer, body positivity activist, kink enthusiast, and pagan, living and creating in Oakland, California. She is devoted to using her performance art and creative works to highlight marginalized peoples. She believes in the beauty of every body, and through the mediums of burlesque and blogging, she breaks down stereotypes and challenges beauty myths to give voice to those silenced by a society that seeks to shame them.

CATHY MILLER is a veteran in the fat liberation community, fighting body oppression since 1976. She has been active in various size-positive organizations for decades, including being coeditor of NAAFA's *Feminist Caucus Newsletter* from 1989 through 1994. She especially enjoyed speaking on body issues to women's studies classes in various local universities. In 1995, Cathy created Big On Batik, an online clothing company exclusively for women of size. For 10 years she created designs and fabrics to delight the eye and adorn beautiful bodies to size 10X. In 2005 she sold the business to a colleague and is now retired, but still active in fighting size oppression.

JEANETTE MILLER is a fierce fat feminist social justice activist, writer/artist, hip-hop addict, and dance floor maven with a penchant for living life boldly and with passion. With an MA in English literature from Portland State

University and an ongoing interest in gender/identity studies, fat studies/activism, and education transformation, she's worked in operations and administration for several public and private universities and also does nonprofit work in an effort to return public education to the public.

LESLEIGH J. OWEN joined the Southern California fat pride movement while researching her dissertation on fat performances and identities. Like the momentum of the movement itself, her participation has only increased until now she feels grateful to know and work with fat pride and fat studies scholars from around the globe. Starting in 2006, Lesleigh has served as a cochair of the Fat Studies Area of the American/Popular Culture Association. Also in 2006, she became a founding member of the Fat Poets' Society, a group that has since published *Fat Poets Speak* and the forthcoming *Fat Poets Speak II*, a collection of fat-themed poems. After receiving her PhD in sociology, Lesleigh became a sociology instructor at Black Hills State University in South Dakota and has published various fat studies articles and even a trashy novel or three.

MONIQA PAULLET is a running enthusiast, secular humanist, and fat acceptance advocate from Dallas, Texas, with a passion for intersectional feminist activism. She holds a BA in journalism: public relations with a minor in social sciences from the University of North Texas, spent 16 months abroad teaching English as a foreign language in South Korea, and now works as a content and copy editor in addition to serving as race director of the Choice 5k, an event benefiting prochoice organizations in North Texas. Her hobbies include fire spinning, photography, belly dancing, obstacle course racing, and blogging.

CAT PAUSÉ is a human development lecturer and fat studies researcher at Massey University in Palmerston North, New Zealand. Her research focuses on the construction, revision, and maintenance of spoiled identities and the effects on health and well-being of marginalized populations (usually fat individuals). Her work has been published in academic journals such as *Human Development, Somatechnics, Feminist Review,* and HERDSA. She also has an edited book, *Queering Fat Embodiment,* in press with Ashgate (UK). Cat has showcased her work on news programs such as *Close Up, Breakfast,* and *20/20,* and regularly contributes to the Australian online journal *The Conversation.* Cat maintains a presence in the Fatosphere through her Tumblr, YouTube channel, podcast, and blog, *Friend of Marilyn.* She may also be found on Twitter, @FOMNZ.

EREC SMITH is an assistant professor of rhetoric and composition at York College of Pennsylvania. Recent publications include "Making Room for Fat Studies in Writing Center Theory and Practice," published in *Praxis: A Writing Center Journal,* and *The Making of Barack Obama: The Rhetoric of Persuasion,* coedited with Matthew Abraham. Smith is both a scholar and activist for size acceptance.

JUANA TANGO was born in a burst of glitter on a radical burlesque stage. She's a fierce advocate of inclusive, diverse, and accessible safe(r) space with more than a decade of social justice, fat acceptance, Latina, queer, and alternative communities experience that reflects both her personal identities and her educational background with an AA in Mexican and Latin American studies and baccalaureate work in community studies with an emphasis on Latina studies.

MARILYN WANN is a longtime fat activist and author of the *FAT!SO?* book as well as a contributor to the *Fat Studies Reader*. She gives weight diversity talks in the United States and internationally. Her original Yay! Scales, which give compliments instead of numbers, are available at the Voluptuart shop online.

JESSICA WILSON is a Health at Every Size registered dietician at My Kitchen Dietitian, LLC, who sees private clients virtually and in person in the San Francisco Bay Area and helps them build healthy and satisfying relationships with food. She has a master's degree in human physiology and years of experience working with Division I athletes. She now applies this to Every Body Move, a collaboration with a personal trainer, exercise physiologist, and HAES therapist, as they build a fitness community for all bodies in the Bay Area.

JULIANNE WOTASIK has been involved in the size acceptance movement since 2007. She is happy to out and proud as a queer, fat-celebrating activist. Her loves in life include her wonderful partner, her horribly spoiled dogs, and her cute pointy hedgehog.

Index